MONOGRAPHS IN PSYCHOBIOLOGY AND DISEASE
Volume 1   Psychobiology of Essential Hypertension

PSYCHOBIOLOGY OF ESSENTIAL HYPERTENSION

Herbert Weiner, M.D.

Montefiore Hospital and Medical Center

ELSEVIER

New York ● Oxford ● Amsterdam

Elsevier North Holland, Inc.
52 Vanderbilt Avenue, New York, New York 10017

Elsevier/North-Holland Biomedical Press
335 Jan Van Galenstraat, P.O. Box 211
Amsterdam, The Netherlands

Modified from chapter 2 of H. Weiner, *Psychobiology and Human Disease.*
Copyright 1977 by Elsevier North Holland, Inc.

Library of Congress Cataloging in Publication Data

Weiner, Herbert M   1921-
    Psychobiology of essential hypertension.
    (Monographs in psychobiology and disease)

    Bibliography: p.
    Includes index.
    1. Hypertension—Psychosomatic aspects. 2. Hypertension—Social aspects.
 3. Psychobiology. I. Title. II. Series. [DNLM: 1. Hypertension—Psychology.
 2. Hypertension—Physiopathology. WG340.3 W423p]
RC685.H8W44   616.1'32'08   79-10969
ISBN 0-444-00275-8

Printed in the United States of America

This book is for
Dora,
Tim, Richard and Tony

CONTENTS

psychological ones. Poor black people (especially men) in the United States are at much greater risk for essential hypertension than are their white compatriots. Salt eating as a personal and cultural habit may play a role in the disease. Behavioral states also affect blood pressure levels, which are much lower in sleep than during the waking state; however, the pattern of BP fluctuations during sleep may be different in hypertensive than in normotensive persons.

Psychological factors appear to play a role either at some stage in the natural history of the disease, or of one of the various subforms of the disease and not in other ones. Psychobiologists in the past have overemphasized the role of these factors in pathogenesis, seemingly unaware that essential hypertension is multifactorial and heterogeneous. Psychological factors clearly do not by *themselves* account for the predisposition to, or pathogenesis of, as complex a disorder as this. The evidence also accumulates that physiological heterogeneity in the initiation of essential hypertension is reflected in psychological heterogeneity. If this contention is supported by more investigation, it would clarify many of the issues that have caused disagreement among psychobiologists working in this area.

At the present time a resurgence of interest in the roles of social and psychological factors in the natural history of this disease can be discerned. Hypertensive patients often do not comply with their prescribed regimens. The various animal models of experimental high blood pressure teach us that the brain participates at some stage or other of the development or maintenance of increased blood pressure levels. The roles on increased sympathetic and decreased parasympathetic discharge in the initiation of some forms of human essential hypertension has again been asserted.

The role of the brain has always been implicit in the psychobiological approach; but because our knowledge of the relationship of mind to brain is still rudimentary, it cannot explicitly be told how experience may alter brain mechanisms that control and regulate the circulation. Only future research will begin to answer this and many related questions. This monograph was written in the hope that it may contribute to the clarification of questions and, therefore, to their answers.

Other monographs in this series will deal with peptic ulcer disease, bronchial asthma, Graves' disease, rheumatoid arthritis, ulcerative colitis and other diseases. All of these diseases are complex and not fully understood: In fact, they are less well understood than is essential hypertension. Because we do not understand them, the assertions that they are multifactorial and heterogeneous are less convincing; yet these diseases are as interesting and enigmatic as is essential hypertension—psychobiological factors also seem to contribute to them.

The monographs on these diseases consist of the individual chapters of a book, published in 1977, entitled *Psychobiology and Human Disease*. They are being made available in monograph form for the reader interested only in certain of these diseases.

PSYCHOBIOLOGY OF ESSENTIAL HYPERTENSION

INTRODUCTION

The text that follows this introduction was written during 1970–1975. Since that time many new studies have been published that attest to the belief that essential hypertension is both heterogeneous and multifactorial. Its heterogeneity manifests itself in two ways: (1) different pathogenetic mechanisms may bring about elevations of blood pressure and (2) different physiological mechanisms may occur at different stages of the natural history of the subforms of essential hypertension. (In fact, there is increasing evidence that the factors that bring about elevations of blood pressure in essential hypertension are different from those that sustain them.) The multifactorial nature of the disease is apparent in that no one factor accounts either for its etiology, pathogenesis or maintenance.

These assertions are emphasized, not because they provide any final solution to the problem of essential hypertension, but because they document a paradigmatic shift in our concepts of disease. No one who reads the massive tome that Genest and his colleagues published in 1977 would conclude that a *single* cause of this disease suffices to explain it. Although the authors of this definitive volume do not provide us with a complete explanation of essential hypertension, they are agreed that there is no simple way of accounting for all its various subforms in the majority of patients.

Essential hypertension has emerged in the 20th century as a disease that is as paradigmatic as the infectious diseases were in the late 19th century. Since Pasteur and Koch, and until very recently, we have lived with very simple explanations of the infectious diseases. But as our knowledge about them grows, such simple explanations no longer

1

suffice—the interactions of a virus and its host are complex and multifactorial (Blumberg, 1977; Gadjusek, 1977; de-Thé et al., 1978). Therefore, the complexity of the etiology, pathogenesis and pathophysiology of essential hypertension should no longer come as a surprise to anyone acquainted with our changing concepts of disease. As Page (1977) has recently written,

> the science of hypertension has too long been slowed by excessive reductionism. Reductionism has been, and always will be, essential, but true understanding of living organisms also requires synthesis. . . .

THE HETEROGENEITY OF BORDERLINE ESSENTIAL HYPERTENSION

There are no established ways of identifying persons at risk for the development of essential hypertension. Two strategies have, therefore, been devised in the past few years: The first is to classify hypertensive patients according to physiological patterns that consist of deviations of cardiac output, plasma renin activity (PRA) or plasma volume (Julius et al., 1975; Laragh et al., 1972; Tarazi et al., 1970). However, these pathophysiological patterns may not necessarily indicate differences in the etiology or pathogenesis of essential hypertension; they might simply reflect a different stage of the disease. For example, high PRA may occur early, or very late in the end stages of the disease. Nevertheless, elevations of PRA in the stages are believed to come about by different mechanisms. The manner of classifying patients does not, however, prove that different forms of essential hypertension exist. The second and the best research strategy available is to study patients very early in the disease process, before (mal)adaptive changes to high blood pressures itself occur. Some of these secondary adaptations consist of a diminution in the sensitivity of the arterial baroreceptors (Korner et al., 1974); an increase in peripheral resistance in response to an increase in cardiac output; structurally increased resistance to regional blood flow (Folkow and Hallbäck, 1977); and changes in cardiac performance (Frohlich et al., 1971).

Other changes in many systems are also found in abiding essential hypertension. To mention just two: Significant increases in the plasma concentration of aldosterone occur with age in essential hypertension in contrast to a decline with age of plasma aldosterone levels in normotensive subjects (Genest et al., 1978); and (as mentioned) PRA is markedly increased during the development of the malignant phase of hypertensive disease and renal failure. Complex changes also occur in renal dynamics that are believed to be the consequence of a subform of the borderline hypertensive state, in which an increased activity of the sympathetic nervous system (and probably diminished parasympathetic activity) occurs. Renal blood flow is reduced by reversible intrarenal vasoconstriction, and increases in circulating norepinephrine and in sympathetic drive both reduce the urinary excretion of sodium and water (Hollenberg and Adams, 1976; Brown et al., 1977). But the rise in BP should cause an increased excretion of sodium and water, which at first does and later does not occur. Therefore, a progressive resetting of the relationship of BP to sodium and water excretion—a regulatory disturbance—is produced. Progressive renal changes ensue to account for the change from borderline labile hypertension to

2

essential hypertension. In short, the BP increases that were initiated elsewhere are maintained by the kidney by a fall in renal blood flow and renin and a rise in total and renal vascular resistance (Brown et al. 1977).

Not all patients with borderline essential hypertension go on to essential hypertension. Groups of patients with borderline hypertension tend to have some increase in cardiac output, increased cardiac contractility and heart rate. Their plasma catecholamine levels are likely to be higher and the urinary excretion of catecholamines is excessive on standing. Stress produces exaggerated catecholamine and BP responses. Ganglionic blocking agents produce a fall in BP that closely correlates with a fall in plasma norepinephrine levels (De Quattro and Miura, 1973; Julius and Esler, 1975; Kuchel, 1977; Lorimer et al., 1971; Louis et al., 1973).

Patients with borderline hypertension differ as a group (but not necessarily as individuals) from normotensive subjects. However, the patients also differ from each other. Not all patients with borderline hypertension have an elevated cardiac output: In 30% the cardiac output is two standard deviations beyond the mean for normal age-matched subjects. In this subgroup of patients, the total peripheral resistance is inappropriately normal at rest (it should be decreased when increased tissue perfusion is brought about by the increased cardiac output). In other patients with borderline hypertension in whom normal cardiac output and heart rate are found, the total peripheral resistance is increased at rest, possibly due to increased alpha-adrenergic vasoconstrictor tone. Blood volume is unevenly distributed in the circulation (mainly in the cardiopulmonary bed) in borderline hypertension, but only in those patients with an increased cardiac output. In about 30% of all patients with borderline hypertension PRA and norepinephrine concentration are elvated. Other patients increase their PRA excessively with postural changes. Yet the increased PRA does not seem to maintain the heightened BP levels through its agency on angiotensin II and aldosterone production. The increased heart rate, cardiac output and PRA can be reduced to normal levels with propranolol, but the plasma norepinephrine concentration and BP continue to remain elevated. Therefore the enhanced PRA is believed to be a result of increased sympathetic activity and is not the primary pathogenetic factor in raising the BP (Esler et al., 1977; Julius and Esler, 1975). (The reverse causal sequence is, however, thought to account for the malignant phase of hypertension when high PRA is found.)

Nonetheless, many borderline hypertensive patients have normal PRA and some have low PRA (Esler et al., 1975). Patients whose PRA is normal tend to be those with diminished stroke volume and cardiac index, normal pulse rate, but increased total peripheral resistance. Their plasma norepinephrine concentration is higher than normal but lower than in patients with high PRA with borderline hypertension. The increased peripheral resistance and BP in patients with borderline hypertension with low or normal PRA is unaffected by the administration of alpha- and beta-adrenergic blocking agents and atropine. The administration of these drugs causes a fall in BP and peripheral resistance in patients with high PRA borderline hypertension (Esler et al., 1975, 1977).

These results suggest that borderline hypertension—a harbinger of established hypertension—is a heterogeneous disturbance with perhaps three different physiological and humoral profiles. These profiles in turn reflect different pathogeneses for borderline hypertension. In fact, endocrine changes in other borderline hypertensive patients are also not completely uniform. (However, these patients may not be the same ones as those who have been studied for their cardiovascular dynamics, their responses to sympathetic and parasympathetic blocking agents and their PRA.) In any case, patients with borderline hypertension can be divided into those whose BP falls below 140/90 mm Hg with reassurance and rest and those in whom no fall occurs (Genest et al., 1978). In both groups of patients a significant mean increase in plasma aldosterone concentration is found; this reverts to normal levels, but only in those who become normotensive. Both groups of patients, when recumbent, show a decreased metabolic clearance rate of aldosterone when compared to normal control subjects. Usually an upright posture considerably decreases the metabolic clearance of aldosterone, but not in patients with mild borderline hypertension. Although other alterations in aldosterone metabolism, binding of the hormone to a specific plasma globulin and responses to stimulation occur in borderline hypertensive patients, the point of this discussion is that borderline patients with mild hypertension are similar in some ways and different in others.

Substance has also been added to the speculation, which appears in the ensuing text, that the physiological heterogeneity of patients with essential hypertension is also reflected in their psychological heterogeneity. Esler and his co-workers (1977) have reported that 16 men, 18–35 years of age, belonging to the subform of borderline hypertensives, in which high PRA and increased plasma norepinephrine levels are found, differ psychologically from 15 borderline hypertensive men with normal PRA and from 20 men with normal blood pressures. The patients with high-renin essential hypertension differ significantly from both the normotensive patients and the hypertensive patients with normal plasma renin activity on a number of psychological measures that signify that they are controlled, guilt-ridden, submissive persons with higher levels of unexpressed or unexpressable anger. But neither hypertensive group scored higher on scores signifying anxiety than did the control groups. The only tendency that differentiated the control group from the hypertensive patients with normal PRA is that they appeared to be more resentful, though as capable of expressing this resentment as were their normotensive peers.

This study documents the psychological heterogeneity of hypertensive patients; it also confirms the psychiatric description of hypertensive patients that we owe to Alexander. Nonetheless, the meaning of this important study is not clear. Julius and Esler (1975) and Esler and colleagues (1977) have argued that the pathogenesis of high-renin borderline hypertension is neurogenic—that the high PRA is secondary to increased sympathetically mediated renin release because the effect of propranolol is to lower PRA but not BP in these patients (Stumpe et al., 1976). They have concluded that in this subform of essential hypertension, either increased sympathetic nervous system activity or both sympathetic nervous system enhancement and diminished parasympathetic inhibition, due to a disturbance in central autonomic regulation, account for their findings. The increased sympathetic nervous system activity would account for all the findings in this subform of essential hypertension.

It would also be enticing to explain the increased sympathetic nervous system activity on the basis of suppressed hostility. However, the findings of Esler and his co-workers are of a correlational nature: The chronically suppressed hostility may not antecede the increased sympathetic drive, it might result from it; perhaps both are the expressions of

4

some altered central nervous system state. Psychosomatic investigators have in the past been guided largely by the concept that suppressed hostility, such as that found by Esler and his co-workers, initiates all forms of hypertension. Clearly, their study does not support this contention—other patients with borderline essential hypertension do not show this psychological trait. Besides, the hostility itself does not explain the pathogenesis of this one form, let alone all forms, of hypertension. Cobb and Rose (1973) found that occupational stress may significantly be related to hypertension. But stressed subjects also develop other diseases besides hypertension; therefore they must be differently predisposed.

The behavior of hypertensive animals also differs from that of normotensive ones. For example, Rifkin et al., (1974) stated that 33-week-old spontaneously hypertensive rats, who already had elevated BPs, were much more likely to kill mice introduced into their cages than were matched normotensive rats. Within the group of hypertensive rats, the rats who committed muricide had more labile BPs and somewhat lower levels than did hypertensive nonkillers.

Again, one may not conclude that muricide in hypertensive rats is causally related to the development of "spontaneous" hypertension; the muricidal behavior should be present before the elevations in BP occur in these animals. We do not know that it is. The approach that should be used is the establishment of a relationship between specific behavior patterns and the predisposition to experimental hypertension, and not to the expression of the disease itself. Haber and her colleagues (1978) have used this strategy. Normotensive salt-sensitive and salt-resistant rats were compared on a number of behavioral measures. Most of the salt-sensitive strain rats were more active and exploratory, especially when older (6 weeks after weaning). Behavioral differences may antecede the development of experimental hypertension in rats, but this would not mean that the relationship is causal; both might be functionally related to altered brain function, which is already manifest in spontaneously hypertensive rats before high BP develops and expresses itself as an increased reactivity to environmental stimuli (Okamoto 1972).

One such central factor may be the brain isorenin system, which is known to produce angiotensins in the brain. An angiotensin-like peptide has been found in the brains of rats with spontaneous hypertension. Isorenin activity increases with brain maturation in some animals. The intraventricular injection of a competitive antagonist of angiotensin lowers BP levels in the spontaneously hypertensive rats, especially after bilateral nephrectomy, suggesting that the brain isorenin—angiotensin system maintains high BP in spontaneously hypertensive rats. In addition, angiotensin levels are known to be high in the cerebrospinal fluid of these rats before they develop high BPs. Angiotensin also excites neurosecretory neurons in the cat's brain and has important interactions with catecholaminergic systems (Ganten et al., 1977; Nicoll and Barker, 1971; Phillips et al., 1977). It is possible, therefore, that both the behavioral state and BP elevations in these rats reflect neurochemical alterations in their brains.

These data strongly support the idea that no single or invariant set of etiological or pathogenetic factors exist in essential hypertension. Yet some authorities still favor one system or the other as the "primary" or fundamental one in its onset—such as an increased or inappropriately high peripheral resistance, or altered intrarenal dynamics. However, the evidence supports the following statements.

5

1. In some patients essential hypertension (e.g., high-renin borderline hypertension) begins with increased sympathetic (and decreased parasympathetic) discharge that leads to elevated plasma catecholamine levels, high PRA and increased cardiac output and heart rate with an inappropriately normal peripheral resistance. A number of maladaptive changes in the baroreceptors, resistance vessels and the kidney ensue to sustain the elevated blood pressure.

2. In other patients with essential hypertension, or those who ingest inordinate amounts of salt, increased peripheral resistance results not from increased sympathetic discharge, but from increased tone, sensitivity and, therefore, responsiveness of the arteriolar smooth muscle either to normal levels of norepinephrine or to angiotensin II and, therefore, aldosterone secretion.

This statement does not exclude the possibility that psychological factors could not play a role in this form of essential hypertension, because ACTH secretion, which is highly responsive to "stress," may in turn stimulate aldosterone secretion.

This form of essential hypertension places the pathogenetic burden either on excessive salt intake or increased mineralocorticoid activity that enhances arteriolar tone and contractility. A biased set of resistance vessels results, upon which many influences—from the psychological to the chemical—may play to enhance peripheral resistance through the medium of norepinephrine, angiotensin II and III and aldosterone. The kidney will later show changes in blood flow with maladaptive changes that result in an altered relationship between the perfusion pressure and sodium and water excretion.

3. In malignant and renovascular hypertension, excessive renin is produced as kidney function is progressively impaired. As a result, angiotensin II levels are high, leading to enhanced aldosterone production and increased sympathetic activity, both of which act on resistance vessels further to increase their resistance to flow (Brown et al., 1977; Genest et al., 1978).

These various models suggest a heterogeneous pathogenesis of essential hypertension and different roles for psychological factors in different forms of the disorder. The evidence grows that it is a disorder of adaptation and regulation. Several regulatory disturbances (in addition to those mentioned) in different systems are known (Genest, 1977; Williams and Dluhy, 1977).

MULTIFACTORIAL NATURE OF ESSENTIAL HYPERTENSION

Many examples of the multifactorial nature of the various forms of essential hypertension exist (Genest, 1977; Herrmann et al., 1976). To ascribe high blood pressure to a single inciting factor, such as a pheochromocytoma, may be an oversimplification. In some but not all patients, pheochromocytomas are associated with elevations of BP despite the fact that the circulating levels of catecholamines are about the same in all. The removal of the tumor does not lower the high BP in all patients (Peart, 1977). Some secondary mechanism, probably renal in origin, sustains the BP in those operated patients who continue to have BP elevations.

Most forms of experimental hypertension in animals are also multifactorial in nature. (Admittedly no consensus has been reached as to whether the various forms of experimental hypertension exactly replicate human essential hypertension.) Nonetheless, animal models of high BP are heuristically powerful; they teach us that multiple factors are involved in raising the BP and that the pathogenesis of high BP is not invariant. For example, the Brookhaven salt-sensitive strain of rat is genetically predisposed to high BP if exposed to a diet high in salt; but when these rats are maintained on a low salt diet (0.4% or 2%NaCl) and exposed for 26 weeks to a chronic, aversive operant conditioning schedule, their BP levels increase. The BP elevation is not as excessive as that produced by a diet containing 4% or 8% of NaCl (Friedman and Iwai, 1977). Therefore, in these genetically predisposed animals different inciting causes—salt feeding or aversive conditioning—may lead to high BP, albeit not to the same degree.

In other closely related animals, the pathogenetic mechanisms differ. In the Milan Wistar strain of spontaneously hypertensive rat the origins of the high BP seem to reside in the kidney (Bianchi et al., 1973, 1974; Folkow and Hallbäck, 1977). By contrast, the primary pathogenetic factors in the Kyoto Wistar strain of spontaneously hypertensive rat appear to reside in the nervous system and are mediated both by its sympathetic outflow and by ACTH and TSH (Okamoto, 1972). Subsequently, changes in the resistance vessels, the kidney and the chemical composition of the heart occur to sustain the high BP (Folkow and Hallack, 1977). However, environmental influences interact with genetic predisposition in these animals: The development of high BP may be slowed by socially isolating very young animals of this strain (Hallbäck, 1975), and may be accelerated by "stress" (Yamori et al., 1969).

These examples illustrate the concept that in animals high BP may have different pathogeneses, and that the inciting factors are different than the sustaining ones. Multiple factors interact. Furthermore, the genetic predisposition to high BP is also heterogeneous, because several different kinds of rat strain with experimental hypertension have now been bred.

Essential hypertension in adolescent persons is also multifactorial: Complex interactions among ethnic origin, socioeconomic status and weight occur. Weight alone accounts for about 20% of the etiological variance of BP levels in adolescents. When BP differences are adjusted for differences due to weight, black adolescents have significantly higher BP levels than their white peers, and black inner-city adolescents have the highest levels. The incidence of systolic BP levels above 140 mm Hg is 10% in black boys, 1% in black girls, and not present at all in white boys and girls in a middle-class school (Kotchen et al., 1974). This study begins to resolve much of the controversy about the results of epidemiological studies in hypertension, because many past studies have only considered a single factor—be it salt intake or socioeconomic status—to account for all of the etiological variance in essential hypertension.

The multifactorial nature of essential hypertension is also entirely in keeping with the data and concept that genetic factors play a role in its etiology. These genetic factors are believed to be polygenic (Pickering, 1968). A polygenic inheritance could account for the fact that several etiological and pathogenetic mechanisms, which otherwise interact in the regulation of BP, deviate quantitatively, not qualitatively, from the norm. In this manner, a number of interactive regulatory deviations may be found in the various subforms of essential hypertension. The search for any one qualitative abnormality, therefore, could be fruitless (Page, 1977).

These quantitative factors—the regulatory disturbances—interact with environmental ones that cause them to be expressed. Among these environmental factors are social and psychological ones. No one would contend today that either one or the other in isolation is the *cause* of essential hypertension (Genest, 1977; Henry and Stephens, 1977). Some psychological traits may interact with physiological ones—for example, increased sympathetic discharge and decreased parasympathetic discharge—early in some forms of borderline hypertension. However, they may play no initiating role in other forms. They may help sustain or aggravate high BP in these forms by a variety of neural and hormonal mediating mechanisms (Zanchetti, 1972).

To quote Page (1977) once again:

> Hypertension under this concept can begin in many ways and also develop in many ways. . . . The theory does not rule out the initiation of hypertension by one stimulus. Experience, however, shows that what appears to be one stimulus usually involves multiple mechanisms ranging from genetic to emotional stress.

REFERENCES

Bianchi, G., Fox, V., and Imbasciati, E. 1974. The development of a new strain of spontaneously hypertensive rats. *Life Sci.* 14:339.
———, ———, DiFrancesco, G. F., Bardi, U., and Radice, M. 1973. Hypertensive role of the kidney in spontaneously hypertensive rats. *Clin. Sci. Mol. Med.* 45 (Suppl. 1):15s.
Blumberg, B. S. 1977. Australia antigen and the biology of hepatitis B. *Science* 197:17.
Brown, J. J., Fraser, R., Lever, A. J., Morton, J. J., Robertson, J. I. S., and Schalekamp, M. A. D. H. 1977. Mechanisms in hypertension: A personal view. In *Hypertension*, edited by J. Genest, E. Koiw and O. Kuchel. New York: McGraw-Hill.
Cobb, S., and Rose, R. M. 1973. Hypertension, peptic ulcer, and diabetes in air traffic controllers. *J. Am Med. Assoc.* 224:489.
de-Thé, G., Geser, A., Day, N. E., Tukei, P. M., Williams, E. H., Beri, D. P., Smith, P. G., Dean, A. G., Bornkamm, G. W., Feorino, P., and Henle, W. 1978. Epidemiological evidence for causal relationship between Epstein–Barr virus and Burkitt's lymphoma from Ugandan prospective study. *Nature* (London) 274:756.
DeQuattro, V., and Miura, Y. 1973. Neurogenic factors in human hypertension: Mechanism or myth? *Am. J. Med.* 55:362.
Esler, M. D., Julius, S., Randall, O. S., Ellis, C. N., and Kashima, T. 1975. Relation of renin status to neurogenic vascular resistance in borderline hypertension. *Am. J. Cardiol.* 36:708.
———, ———, Zweifler, A., Randall, O., Harburg, E., Gardiner, H., and DeQuattro, V. 1977. Mild high-renin essential hypertension. *N. Engl. J. Med.* 296:405.
Folkow, B. U. G., and Hallbäck, M. I. L. 1977. Physiopathology of spontaneous hypertension in rats. In *Hypertension*, edited by J. Genest, E. Koiw and O. Kuchel. New York: McGraw-Hill.
Friedman, R., and Iwai, J. 1977. Dietary sodium, psychic stress and genetic predisposition to experimental hypertension. *Proc. Soc. Exp. Med. Biol.* 155:449.

Frohlich, E. D., Tarazi, R. C., and Dustan, H. P. 1971. Clinical—physiological correlation in the development of hypertensive heart disease. *Circulation* 44:446.

Gadjusek, D. C. 1977. Unconventional viruses and the origin and disappearance of Kuru. *Science* 197:943.

Ganten, D., Schelling, P., and Ganten, U. 1977. Tissue isorenins. In *Hypertension,* edited by J. Genest, E. Koiw, and O. Kuchel. New York: McGraw-Hill.

Genest, J. 1977. Basic mechanisms of essential hypertension. In *Hypertension,* edited by J. Genest, E. Koiw and O. Kuchel. New York: McGraw-Hill.

———, Koiw, E., and Kuchel, O. 1977. *Hypertension.* New York: McGraw-Hill.

———, Nowaczynski, W., Boucher, R., and Kuchel, O. 1978. Role of the adrenal cortex and sodium in the pathogenesis of human hypertension. *Can. Med. Assoc. J.* 118:538.

Haber, S. B., Friedman, R., and Iwai, J. 1978. The relationship between genotype and behavior in experimental hypertension. Submitted for publication.

Hallbäck, M. I. L. 1975. Consequences of social isolation on blood pressure, cardiovascular reactivity and design in spontaneously hypertensive rats. *Acta Physiol. Scand.* 93:455.

Henry, J. P., and Stephens, P. M. 1977. *Stress, Health, and the Social Environment: A Sociobiological Approach to Medicine.* New York: Springer-Verlag.

Herrmann, H. J. M., Rassek, M., Schäfer, N., Schmidt, Th., and von Uexküll, Th. 1976. Essential hypertension—Problems, concepts and an attempted synthesis. In *Modern Trends in Psychosomatic Medicine—3,* edited by O. W. Hill. London: Butterworths.

Hollenberg, N. K., and Adams, D. F. 1976. The renal circulation in hypertensive disease. *Am. J. Med.* 60:773.

Julius, S., and Esler, M. 1975. Autonomic nervous cardiovascular regulation in borderline hypertension. *Am. J. Cardiol.* 36:685.

———, Randall, O. S., Esler, M. D., Kashima, T., Ellis, C. N., and Bennett, J. 1975. Altered cardiac responsiveness and regulation in the normal cardiac output type of borderline hypertension. *Circ. Res.* 36—37 (Suppl. 1):199.

Korner, P. I., West, M. J., Shaw, J., and Uther, J. B. 1974. "Steady state" properties of the baroreceptor—heart rate reflex in essential hypertension in man. *Clin. Exp. Pharmacol. Physiol.* 1:65.

Kotchen, J. M., Kotchen, T. A., Schwertman, N. C., and Kuller, L. H. 1974. Blood pressure distributions of urban adolescents. *Am. J. Epidemiol.* 99:315.

Kuchel, O. 1977. Autonomic nervous system in hypertension: Clinical aspects. In *Hypertension,* edited by J. Genest, E. Koiw and O. Kuchel. New York: McGraw-Hill.

Laragh, J. H., Baer, L. H., Brunner, H. R., Bühler, F. R., Sealey, J. E., and Vaughan, E. D., Jr. 1972. Renin, angiotensin and aldosterone in pathogenesis and management of hypertensive vascular disease. *Am. J. Med.* 52:633.

Lorimer, A. R., McFarlane, P. W., Provan, G., Duffy, T., and Lawrie, T. D. V. 1971. Blood pressure and catecholamine responses to stress in normotensive and hypertensive subjects. *Cardiovasc. Res.* 5:169.

Louis, W. J., Doyle, A. E., Anavekar, S. N., and Chua, K. G. 1973. Sympathetic activity and essential hypertension. *Clin. Sci. Mol. Med.* 45:1195.

Nicoll, R. A., and Barker, J. L. 1971. Excitation of supraoptic neurosecretory cells by angiotensin II. *Nat. New Biol.* 233:172.

Okamoto, K. 1972. *Spontaneous Hypertension.* Tokyo: Igaku Shoin.

Page, I. H. 1977. Some regulatory mechanisms of renovascular and essential hypertension. In *Hypertension,* edited by J. Genest, E. Koiw and O. Kuchel. New York: McGraw-Hill.

Peart, W. S. 1977. Personal views on mechanisms of hypertension. In *Hypertension,* edited by J. Genest, E. Koiw and O. Kuchel. New York: McGraw-Hill.

Phillips, M. I., Mann, J. F. E., Haebara, H., Dietz, R., Schelling, P., and Ganten, D. 1977. Lowering of hypertension by central saralasin in the absence of plasma renin. *Nature* (London) 270:445.

Pickering, G. 1968. *High Blood Pressure.* London: J. & A. Churchill.

Rifkin, R. J., Silverman, J. M., Chavez, F. T., and Frankl, G. 1974. Intensified mouse killing in the spontaneously hypertensive rat. *Life Sci.* 14:985.

Stumpe, K. O., Kolloch, R., Vetter, H., Gramman, W., Krück, F., Ressel, Ch., and Higuchi, M. 1976. Acute and long-term studies of the mechanisms of action of beta-blocking drugs in lowering blood pressure. *Am. J. Med.* 60:853.

Tarazi, R. C., Dustan, H. P., Frohlich, E. D., Gifford, R. W., Jr., and Hoffman, G. C. 1970. Plasma volume and chronic hypertension. Relationship to arterial pressure levels in different hypertensive diseases. *Arch. Intern. Med.* 125:835.

Williams, G. H., and Dluhy, R. G. 1977. Regulation of renin—angiotensin—aldosterone axis in hypertension. In *Hypertension,* edited by J. Genest, E. Koiw and O. Kuchel. New York: McGraw-Hill.

Yamori, Y., Matsumoto, M., Yamabe, H., and Okamoto, K. 1969. Augmentation of spontaneous hypertension by chronic stress in rats. *Jap. Circ. J.* 33:399.

Zanchetti, A. 1972. Neural factors and catecholamines in experimental hypertension. In *Neural and Psychological Mechanisms in Cardiovascular Disease,* editged by A. Zanchetti. Milan: Il Ponte.

Zweifler, A. J., and Esler, M. 1976. Dissociation of fall in blood pressure, renin activity and heart rate during propranolol therapy. *Circulation* 54:87.

Essential hypertension and the complications it produces constitute the major hazard to the health of the members of most Western societies. Because it ravages health, and because its pathophysiology is complex and interesting, it has received more investigative attention than any other disease. Despite the vast variety of studies on the factors that control blood pressure and the multiple variables that regulate the circulation and the excretion of salt and water, no agreement has been reached as to which factors elevate blood pressure levels. The regulation of blood pressure and of the circulation, of salt, water and extracellular fluid volume constitutes one of the marvels of Nature. Innumerable processes in intimate interaction regulate them; some processes are self-regulatory, others are influenced by multiple and complex inputs at several levels of organization. Although much is known about these processes both in health and in essential hypertension, no definitive data or theory satisfactorily accounting for the disease has been presented.

Many regulatory processes maintain blood pressure levels within a remarkably narrow range in human beings at rest. Admittedly, blood pressure levels vary a great deal within this range with changes in posture and salt intake, with exercise, heat, cold, noise, pain, emotional and sexual excitement, mental concentration, novel situations, and during

Some sections of this chapter originally appeared in a different version in *Psychosomatics in Essential Hypertension*, eds. M. Koster, H. Musaph, and P. Visser under the title, "Psychosomatic Research in Essential Hypertension: Retrospect and Prospect." Reprinted here with permission of the publisher. Copyright 1970 by S. Karger AG, Basel.

talking. Blood pressure levels also tend to rise with age in most human beings. Blood pressure levels vary within a certain range not only with changes in the environment or with age, but with changes in the behavioral state of human beings: blood pressure levels may either be highly variable or be at very low levels (60/40 mm Hg) in sleeping adults. On awakening, the blood pressure rises to levels within the normal range.

Once resting blood pressure levels rise above some arbitrary level—140/90 mm Hg, for example—the physician suspects essential hypertension, especially if the levels remain above this level on repeated measurement. Presumably, one or other of the many mechanisms that maintain the blood pressure within the usual range have failed.

The problem of essential hypertension is so complex that we may well be at the very limits of our capacity to account for and conceptualize the multiple processes involved in its etiology. Our capacity to solve the problem of its etiology is diminished by the fact that there is no established way of discovering who is at risk for this disease. By the time we study patients after the onset of high blood pressure, a set of compensatory physiological processes have set in. It becomes impossible then to differentiate the antecedent initiating factors from the consequent sustaining factors of elevated blood pressure.

In the past 25 years we have also learned that high blood pressure and essential hypertension are not synonymous. Elevations of blood pressure occur in a wide variety of conditions and diseases. They may occur with increased intracranial pressure, various kidney diseases, coarctation of the aorta, renal artery stenosis, aldosterinomas, reninomas, pheochromocytomas, in women taking contraceptive pills, and in Cushing's and Graves' Disease. Although this list is not all-inclusive, it suggests that high blood pressure levels can occur for a variety of reasons, and that high blood pressure should not be used as a synonym for essential hypertension. As our knowledge of this disease increases, new forms of high blood pressure are continually being discovered in patients who are now diagnosed as having "essential" hypertension. At the present time, essential hypertension is probably a heterogeneous disease made up of several unspecified subgroups.

BASIC METHODOLOGICAL AND CONCEPTUAL ISSUES

Problems of Definition

There is general agreement about only three aspects of essential hypertension. The disease consists of an elevation of blood pressure; an increase in peripheral resistance occurs at some time during the course of the disease; and genetic factors play an etiological role in most instances of the disease. There is disagreement about every other aspect of its etiology and pathogenesis. The main, if not the only, reason for this disagreement is that we have no recognized way of predicting who will develop essential hypertension and cannot determine the sequence of events that lead up to it. Several attempts to study patients at risk for the disease have been made. Some adolescents and young adults with a verified family history of hypertension or high blood pressure may be predisposed to develop hypertension later in life (Remington et al., 1960). Other young people have high casual blood pressure levels. Harris et al. (1953), Kalis et al. (1961), and Sokolow and Harris (1961a) showed that college students with high casual pressures differed in

12

psychological functioning from people with lower pressures. Also, in the former, stressful life events produced larger sympathetically mediated vasopressor responses, which lasted longer than in the latter.

Doyle and Fraser (1961) infused norepinephrine into the brachial arteries of the normotensive adult sons of patients with documented essential hypertension and compared them with medical students and house officers of similar ages whose parents did not have elevated blood pressure levels. Norepinephrine was infused into one brachial artery at two different dosage levels—0.2 and 0.4μg per min. The response to infusion was measured in terms of the percent fall in forearm blood flow. At both dose levels the mean responses of the sons of hypertensive parents were significantly greater than those of the sons of normotensive parents. An inherently greater vascular reactivity to norepinephrine infusion is present in the sons of hypertensive parents. This vascular hyperreactivity resides in the smooth muscle of the arteriolar or arterial wall, and may be an inherited trait.

But we do not know whether young people with a high casual blood pressure level or hyperreactive arterioles develop essential hypertension. Essential hypertension is usually diagnosed by chance. The early stage of the disease is asymptomatic. Therefore the task of identifying a population of subjects with essential hypertension remains extremely difficult, as the physician cannot tell when the blood pressure becomes elevated.

The upper limits of normal blood pressure levels are defined arbitrarily; no consensus has been achieved. Pickering (1961) has drawn attention to the lack of agreement about the dividing line between a normal and elevated blood pressure. The dividing line is 120/80 mm Hg in some studies (Robinson and Brucer, 1939) and 180/110 mm Hg in others (Evans, 1920). Most clinicians would consider a blood pressure of 180/110 mm Hg high. Some do not. The dividing line between a normal and high blood pressure is arbitrary and fixed. But blood pressure levels vary continually and markedly throughout the day and night in both hypertensive and normal subjects. Daily measurements of blood pressure may vary by 25 percent or more in patients with initial arterial pressure readings of 140/90 mm Hg (Glock et al., 1957; Koster, 1970). At one time a marked variability in blood pressure levels in normotensive persons was thought to be predictive of future essential hypertension. This method of selecting a population of normotensive patients at risk for essential hypertension has been discredited (Page, 1960). Provocative tests, such as the cold pressor test, or the administration of tetraethylammonium chloride, epinephrine, or norepinephrine (designed to bring out the excessive blood pressure reactivity of the future hypertensive), produce different results in the hands of different investigators. Blood pressure lability by itself cannot be considered to be a reliable predictor of the tendency to develop essential hypertension.

Problems of Diagnosis

It is difficult to establish that the patients who comprise a research sample actually suffer from essential hypertension, and not from one of the gamut of diseases in which high blood pressure is a symptom. This problem can be illustrated by the attempts that have been made to discriminate between primary (Conn's syndrome) and secondary aldosteronism, which are both accompanied by high blood pressure.

Primary aldosteronism may or may not be a very rare cause of symptomatic hypertension. If rare, it does not constitute a problem in the selection of hypertensive subjects for study. But it may be common. In a series of 33 patients with a diagnosis of essential hypertension (Conn et al., 1966), five were found to be normokalemic and to have suppressed plasma renin levels and increased aldosterone production levels. In this series of patients initially diagnosed as having essential hypertension the incidence of Conn's syndrome was 15 percent. Laragh and his co-workers (1966) and Ledingham et al. (1967) concluded from a study of 113 patients with essential hypertension that Conn's syndrome is rare. The lack of agreement about the incidence of Conn's syndrome is due to the difficulty in applying consistent criteria in the diagnosis of primary aldosteronism (Conn et al., 1966; Dollery et al., 1959; Ledingham et al., 1967; Page and McCubbin, 1965).

If primary aldosteronism is as common as Conn and co-workers (1966) believe, differentiating primary aldosteronism from the secondary form poses a major problem in subject selection. When Conn's syndrome (1955) is fully developed— with tetany, weakness, paralysis, high blood pressure, hypokalemia, an excess production of aldosterone, and an adrenal adenoma—it can be distinguished from essential hypertension. In less-blatant or asymptomatic forms of primary aldosteronism, hypokalemia might be variable and mild (Conn et al., 1964). Secondary aldosteronism occurs in malignant and renovascular hypertension and consists of a syndrome of hypokalemia, increased aldosterone production (secondary to increased angiotensin activity) and a high blood pressure (Conn, 1961; Dollery et al., 1959; Laidlaw et al., 1960).

When hypertensive disease is advanced, severe, or long-standing, carbohydrate intolerance may also occur (Biglieri et al., 1967; Christiansen et al., 1964; Kirkendall et al., 1964), presumably as a result of secondary aldosteronism. Aberrations of carbohydrate metabolism are also seen in primary aldosteronism (Conn, 1955; Conn et al., 1966). Many patients with benign essential hypertension have low serum or plasma renin levels (Brunner et al., 1972; Creditor and Loschky, 1967; Gunnels et al., 1967; Ledingham et al., 1967) and their aldosterone secretion is normal.

Primary and secondary aldosteronism can be differentiated, but care is needed. In the secondary form, plasma renin levels are very high (Genest et al., 1964; Morris, 1962). In primary aldosteronism renin levels are either normal or very low (Conn, 1955; Conn et al., 1964; Genest et al., 1964; Meyer, 1967). Many hypertensive patients restrict the amount of salt in their food. A low intake of salt and an upright posture stimulate plasma renin activity (Conn et al., 1964). Care must, therefore, be taken when measurements of renin activity are made in hypertensive patients not to stimulate renin production and simulate primary aldosteronism. Primary and secondary aldosteronism need to be differentiated if an investigator wishes to study some aspect of essential hypertension. Diagnostic difficulties also face the investigator in differentiating between patients with essential and renovascular hypertension.

Conceptual Issues

Conceptual disagreements about a variety of issues characterize hypertension research. To begin with, it is not clear whether an elevated level of blood pressure is but the outward sign of some more basic disturbance, a central feature of the disease, or a normal variation and not a manifestation of disease.

Platt (1967) has argued that blood pressure readings are discontinuously (bimodally) distributed in populations of human beings. Those with high levels of blood pressure are set apart from those with normal levels. High blood pressure levels are, therefore, a manifestation of the disease essential hypertension. Pickering (1967) asserts that blood pressure levels are continuously (unimodally) distributed in the population. At one end of a unimodal or Gaussian distribution of blood pressure, high levels would occur. Therefore, the high blood pressure levels of essential hypertension are due to normal variation, and do not constitute a disease per se.

Pickering's argument disturbs our traditional concepts of disease, for the following reasons. Although essential hypertension is frequently a symptomless disease, persons with essential hypertension are at risk for a number of serious complications from which they die (Bechgaard, 1967). One serious and direct complication of essential hypertension is arterial and arteriolar disease. Since the introduction of arterial surgery for relief of a coarctation of the aorta, it has been found that the sudden impact of elevated blood pressure on the arterial bed distal to the former constriction leads to swelling and necrosis of arterial walls to the point of gangrene (Benson and Sealy, 1956). When blood pressure levels are kept low after surgery the damage is averted (Groves and Effler, 1960). In essential hypertension, arterial lesions often occur after many years of elevated blood pressure levels. Any part of the arterial bed can be affected. In view of the fact that the high blood pressure levels of essential hypertension predispose to arterial damage, it would be hard to argue that it is not a disease.

Patients with "high normal" pressure or "borderline hypertension" are more likely to develop elevated blood pressure levels than are normotensive persons and are, therefore, at risk for arterial disease (Evans, 1957; Hines, 1940; Julius et al., 1964; Julius and Shork, 1970; Palmer, 1930). Twelve percent of persons whose blood pressure readings were initially normal had blood pressure levels of 150/90 mm Hg or more 20 years later. By comparison, 26 percent of those whose blood pressure was more than 140/90 at 20 years of age later had a blood pressure above 150/90 mm Hg (Julius et al., 1964). Therefore, the risk of essential hypertension is doubled in those with borderline high blood pressure at 20 years of age. The risk of dying of the complications of high blood pressure is greater in those with borderline hypertension than in people with normal blood pressure readings (Heyden et al., 1969; Kannel et al., 1969; Levy et al., 1945; Lew, 1967; McKenzie and Shepherd, 1937; Thomson, 1950). And the eventual morbidity for coronary artery disease (Kannel et al., 1969) and other kinds of cardiovascular disease is enhanced in borderline hypertension (Heyden et al., 1969; Thomson, 1950). It is, therefore, difficult to argue that essential hypertension is not a disease, because it does cause death and disability.

The concept that hypertension is "essential," may also be seriously misleading. This label is intended to set essential hypertension apart from kidney diseases or diseases of the endrocrine system in which the etiology and pathogenesis of the blood pressure elevations are better known. The term "essential" implies that we do not know what produces the high blood pressure in essential hypertension (Shapiro, 1973). Actually, more is known than is conceded. The problem is that there is no agreement about what is known. The lack of agreement stems from the need to find a single "cause" for the etiology and pathogenesis of essential hypertension. Single pathogenetic hypotheses are advocated. Some advocate specific defects within the kidney. Others advocate a disturbance in salt intake and metabolism. Still others believe that the adrenal gland is at fault; among them, some point a finger at the adrenocortical hormones, others at the adrenomedullary hormones (norepinephrine). Environmental stresses and the emotional responses that they elicit in physiologically and psychologically predisposed persons have also been blamed for the pathogenesis of essential hypertension. For many years increases in the peripheral resistance were considered to be the antecedent and central "cause" of essential hypertension. And indeed the peripheral resistance is usually elevated in patients with essential hypertension.

Recently, the role of the circulation in the pathogenesis of essential hypertension has been reassessed. It appears that early in the course of essential hypertension in some patients, the cardiac output is elevated, and this in turn later increases the peripheral resistance (Guyton and Coleman, 1969). Therefore, in some patients increases in peripheral resistance are secondary and probably help to sustain, but do not initiate, the development of high blood pressure levels.

These disagreements about the pathogenesis of essential hypertension could be resolved if it could be demonstrated that there is no single invariant "cause" or combination of antecedent causes of this disease. Given the number of variables that control and regulate the arterial pressure, it should not be surprising that elevated levels of blood pressure are produced by a variety of factors that either alter the relationship between these variables or alter the level of one of the variables to bias the entire system. It is now fairly clear that essential hypertension occurs with high, normal, or low renin levels (Brunner et al., 1972). Different mechanisms may, therefore, initiate the disease. No one cause or mechanism does so. Also, it may be important to separate out the mechanisms that initiate the disease from those that sustain it (later in this chapter the reasons for this statement will be described). The disagreements about its pathogenesis could be resolved with studies of subjects at risk for essential hypertension, because once hypertension has begun, it is impossible to determine which devices are involved in initiating the illness and which in sustaining it.

THE CURRENT STATUS OF PSYCHOSOMATIC RESEARCH ON ESSENTIAL HYPERTENSION

The problem of defining essential hypertension and the conceptual issue of attempting to infer its etiology and pathogenesis after onset have also plagued the behavioral scientist. Some behavioral scientists have found that hypertensive patients struggle against unconscious feelings of rage, hatred, and anger. Other behavioral scientists have described the way hypertensive patients perceive other people as dangerous, derisive, unsympathetic, and untrustworthy. Some hypertensive patients, therefore, avoid other people, provoke others to behave in the very manner in which they perceive them, or deny derisive or unsympathetic behavior on the part of others.

Originally, some behavioral scientists believed that the origin of the anger and rage that colors the hypertensive's perceptions could be traced back to frustrated dependency wishes in childhood. More recently, medical sociologists have pointed out that the incidence and prevalence of essential hypertension is highest in the male black population living in the poorest parts of American cities. In that setting, people are particularly liable to experience violence and prejudice, police brutality, economic hardship, family discord, and divorce. The rage that these attitudes and events engender and the alertness to derision and danger are real. Other hypertensive patients struggle against their anger and are afraid to express it. They are often unassertive. Still other patients are assertive, combative, bitter, and rebellious. Most behavioral scientists would agree that many, but not all, hypertensive patients have conflicts about anger and rage that are expressed in different traits, styles, and ways of relating. Probably not all such patients are constituted psychologically in a uniform way.

Even if the psychological characteristics of these patients were uniform, they might not have etiological or pathogenetic significance. Because these characteristics are observed after the onset of the disease, they might be a product of high blood pressure levels or high serum renin and angiotensin activity. Or they might covary with changes in blood pressure levels, sustain them, or influence the course of the disease. Normal or high blood pressure levels do indeed vary markedly throughout the day and night, with everyday events, and with changes in the behavioral state of human beings (Sokolow et al., 1970).

Behavioral and physiological studies on animals strongly suggest that social isolation early in life that is followed by a return to communal life is not only marked by aggressive behavior but results in high blood pressure. On the other hand, genetic factors play a major role in some strains of rats that can be bred for salt sensitivity or the "spontaneous" development of hypertension.

Even if anger and aggression play a role in essential hypertension in man, not all angry people develop it. Anger must be combined with physiological predispositions to the disease. Although the predisposing physiological factors are not known, they seem to consist of a variety of different disturbances in the regulation of blood pressure. Recent studies in animals also point to the fact that the brain participates either in the initiation or in the mediation of the initial phases of experimental hypertension, and it may also be involved in sustaining some other forms of hypertension—a generalization that has always been implicit in the psychosomatic theory of essential hypertension (Alexander, 1950; Charvat et al., 1964; Folkow, 1971; Henry and Cassel, 1969; Weiner, 1970).

THE ROLE OF GENETIC FACTORS IN ESSENTIAL HYPERTENSION

Introduction

Even though no consensus has been reached about the pathogenesis of essential hypertension, genetic factors are believed to play an etiological role in the disease. Essential hypertension is believed to be an inherited disease (Hamilton et al., 1954, 1963; Hoobler, 1961; Pickering, 1955). This belief is based on family and twin studies (Ayman, 1934; Bøe et al., 1957; Hines et al., 1957; Mathers et al., 1961) and the stable incidence of essential hypertension in white persons from Norway to Nassau (Bøe et al., 1957; Johnson and Remington; 1961). The best evidence that genetic factors play a role in high blood pressure comes from animal studies. At least in one strain of rats, the inheritance of high blood pressure is polygenic. It is easier to determine the mode of inheritance by breeding rats than by population studies. Population studies, with few exceptions, do not reveal the mode of inheritance of a trait (McKusick, 1960). Nonetheless, Pickering (1961, 1967) believes that the mode of inheritance of essential hypertension is polygenic. He bases his inference on the fact that he and others (Bøe et al., 1957; Comstock, 1957; Ostfeld and Paul, 1963) have found that the frequency distribution of blood pressure in a population is unimodal. He believes that a particular level of blood pressure is polygenically inherited. In his opinion each of the multiple genetic factors operate through different mechanisms to determine blood pressure levels.

Platt (1947; 1963; 1967) has disagreed with Pickering. He points out that systolic blood pressure is not continuously, but is bimodally (or multimodally) distributed in the population. This distribution speaks for the existence of two or more different populations. The bimodal distribution is also evidence of the existence of a single dominant genetic factor in the etiology of essential hypertension. Platt argues that the two populations might behave differently in regard to increases in blood pressure. In one population a rise in diastolic blood pressure would be expected to occur in middle life. In the other population, very little change in blood pressure would occur at this age. Platt believes that the rise in blood pressure is an inherited trait and not merely a function of age. However, the evidence in support of this thesis (Cruz-Coke, 1959, 1960; Thomson, 1950) is not conclusive.

Pickering (1967) does not consider the rate with which blood pressure levels increase with age to be an inherited trait. Rather he ascribes the increase in blood pressure with age to environmental factors. Pickering's view is indirectly supported by Harris' and Singer's (1968) prospective study of 500 persons working in an insurance company, who were observed for 30 years. The blood pressure of some did not increase at all with age. In some others a steep increase occurred. The increases were continuously distributed throughout this population. If Platt's hypothesis were correct, a majority of subjects would have shown no increase in blood pressure with age, and a few would have developed elevated levels rapidly.

Different populations of both sexes at different ages differ greatly in regard to the rate of change in blood pressure with age (Henry and Cassel, 1969). In some groups (e.g., Navajo Indians on reservations, U.S. Navy aviators, and some rural Africans and Asians) no increase in blood pressure with age occurs. In other groups, such as black persons living in the Southern United States, the rise is steep and begins early in life. The data support Pickering's position that increases in blood pressure are not inherited but indicate the operation of various environmental factors. The data are consistent enough to indicate that genetic factors alone do not account for elevated levels in blood pressure. They also suggest that blood pressure levels are randomly distributed in a population in the same manner as height and weight. In some persons in the population, a tendency to high blood pressure is probably polygenically inherited. This unspecified tendency accounts for about 30 percent of the etiological variance. The tendency is elicited by environmental factors. Some persons with this tendency respond to environmental factors either with high blood pressure levels or essential hypertension. At least in some animals the level of the blood pressure is not inherited; it can be "set" by external factors such as salt or "stress."

Evidence Derived from Studies on Human Twins

Hines et al. (1957) studied the blood pressure levels of 17 monozygotic (Mz) and 3 dizygotic (Dz) twins. Zygosity was determined in 13 twin pairs. Eight pairs of Mz twins were condordant for hypertension. In two of these the hypertension was due to polycystic disease of the kidney. The blood pressure levels in the female twin pairs were concordant. Male Mz twins were concordant for blood pressure levels but discordant for the presence of hypertensive vascular changes. Three Mz twin pairs were discordant for hypertension. Six other Mz pairs were normotensive. 200 additional pairs of twins were studied. Exact zygosity determinations on these twins were not carried out. Of these pairs, 87 were assumed to be Mz. Of the 200 twin pairs, 97 percent were less than 25 years of age: none had hypertension. The blood pressure levels of the Mz twins were more alike in the Dz twins with respect to resting levels and to pressor responses to the cold pressor test. Hines concludes that a "genetic" factor is responsible for the mechanisms that control blood pressure in normotensive and hypertensive persons.

In normotensive male Mz twins the blood pressure variance is greater than in Dz male twins. In female twins the reverse is true in regard to systolic and mean blood pressure. When intrapair variance of blood pressure in male and female Mz twins is compared, the variance in men is consistently larger for systolic blood pressure. Therefore, the basal blood pressure in men is subject to greater environmental influences than in women (Mathers et al., 1961).

Much can be learned from studying Mz twins discordant for blood pressure levels or for essential hypertension in order to determine the factors that are responsible for the different phenotypes. Among these factors may be the psychological state of each of the twins at the time the blood pressure is determined. Instances of essential hypertension developing in the more emotionally disturbed member of four twin pairs have been described (Flynn et al., 1950; Friedman and Kasanin, 1943; Jones et al., 1948; Sheldon and Ball, 1950). Torgersen and Kringlen (1971) studied the blood pressure levels of 48 adult Mz twins. They found that the more obedient, quiet, reserved, submissive, insecure, depressed, and withdrawn of each pair of twins had higher systolic blood pressure levels than his brother or sister. The systolic blood pressure levels in some instances ranged from 97 to 227 mm Hg.

Evidence for Genetic Factors from Studies of Families

The oral contraceptive pills produce elevations of blood pressure only in women with a family history of high blood pressure (Shapiro, 1973). "The pill" presumably elicits a genetically determined tendency to high blood pressure. But this tendency does not account for the finding that spouses, who are not related to each other except by marriage, tend to share similar blood pressure levels the longer they remain married to each other (Winkelstein et al., 1966).* Other family members besides spouses share common blood pressure levels. The family incidence of hypertension is frequent. O'Hare et al. (1924) found a positive family history in almost three-quarters of 300 persons with hypertension. If one parent is hypertensive, 12 to 28 percent of the children also are.

* This finding has not been confirmed by Gearing et al. (1962) and Johnson et al. (1965).

With two hypertensive parents 16 to 41 percent of the children are hypertensive. Of the adult siblings of hypertensive patients, 20 to 65 percent are also hypertensive (Thomas and Cohen, 1955). By comparison, the incidence of hypertension in the siblings of normotensive people is between 6.5 and 20 percent and the incidence is 6 percent in the children of normotensive parents (Johnson et al., 1965; Miall et al., 1962, 1967; Speranksy et al., 1959). Zinner and his co-workers (1971) found that the variation of systolic and diastolic blood pressure levels in children of the same families was less than in unrelated people. Systolic and diastolic blood pressure levels cluster in siblings and their mothers. A family tendency to similar blood pressure levels is established early in life.

The family aggregation of hypertensive and normotensive blood pressure levels is a well-established fact (Perera et al., 1961; Pickering, 1961; Schweitzer et al., 1967) but its interpretation is not, because either genetic or familial factors could acount for the similarity of the blood pressure that occurs in relatives. The similarity of blood pressure levels in families and Mz twins suggests that the level is an inherited trait. Some would disagree with this interpretation. They would consider that a predisposition to high blood pressure is inherited, but the level is not. Another possibility is that dietary factors, such as a sensitivity to salt, are inherited. Studies in hypertensive rats suggest that different physiological mechanisms, including salt sensitivity, may be inherited and may produce high blood pressure levels. Therefore, different genetic factors can be assumed to control different mechanisms that produce high blood pressure levels in rats. And, the search for an invariant set of genetic factors may be fruitless.

The discussions about the inheritance of high blood pressure or of essential hypertension tend to overlook the possibility that it is a heterogeneous illness with different predispositions and initiating factors that are under different genetic control. Support for this suggestion derives from the fact that essential hypertension may occur with low, normal, or high renin levels. And low-renin hypertension can result from different disturbances in the regulation of the renin-angiotensin-aldosterone system that may be inherited (Brunner et al., 1971, 1972).

EPIDEMIOLOGICAL STUDIES OF ESSENTIAL HYPERTENSION

About 70 percent of the etiology of essential hypertension can be accounted for by environmental factors. But environmental factors can be specified only when accurate incidence and prevalence figures for the disease are available—a goal that has not yet been achieved.

Prevalence figures for essential hypertension should be separately gathered for the borderline or early, and the established forms of essential hypertension. Borderline systolic blood pressure elevations occur in about 10 percent of a population of 20 years of age or more. The prevalence of essential hypertension usually increases with age. By the age of 60, its prevalence is 40 percent. Below the age of 50 years it occurs with less prevalence in women than in men. All prevalence figures should, therefore, take into account the sex and age of patients and the specific stage of their disease. Because many studies have failed adequately to classify their subjects along these lines, the large literature on the epidemiology of essential hypertension and high blood pressure is confusing. The incidence and prevalence figures vary from patient series to patient series, according to their age, sex, geographic location and ethnic group. Prevalence figures for the disease vary from 5 to 25 percent or more of a population. Scotch (1961) found an even larger prevalence in South Africa, where it was 20 percent under the age of 45 years and 58 percent in older Zulu men.

There is sound evidence that geographic and cultural factors, in addition to the age and the sex, significantly influence the prevalence of essential hypertension. Natives of New Guinea who live in very "primitive" conditions have higher blood pressure levels (Whyte, 1958) than some Brazilian Indians who live under similar conditions (Loewenstein, 1961). The blood pressures of Indian workers living and working in the tea plantations of Assam (Wilson, 1958) rise with age much more rapidly than in three other Indian populations (Padmavati and Gupta, 1959). Marked differences in the prevalence and the increase of blood pressure levels with age have been observed in various Micronesian societies, whose members live under similar climactic conditions (Lovell, 1967).

In the United States, people who live in towns have higher blood pressure levels (Berkson et al., 1960; Stamler et al., 1967a, b) or mortality rates (Stamler et al., 1967b) than those who live in the country. In black American women an opposite trend is found: in Mississippi, black rural women have higher mean systolic and diastolic blood pressures than black urban women (Langford et al., 1968). Stamler et al. (1967a) reports that the age-corrected prevalence rates per 1,000 men of diastolic blood pressure levels over 95 mm Hg were 209, 108, and 67 in black, native-born white, and foreign-born white blue-collar men in Illinois respectively.

Consistent trends in the prevalence rates of high blood pressure levels are found when black and white Americans are compared. Throughout the United States, black Americans have higher levels (Stamler et al., 1967b). In Detroit, higher blood pressure levels occur in black men living in areas of the city marked by low socioeconomic status, high crime rates, police brutality and high rates of separation and divorce. The blood pressure levels were higher than in the poor blacks than in black or white persons living in areas of the city that were not marked by such social and economic conditions (Harburg et al., 1973). However, differences in blood pressure levels between black and white American women matched for socioeconomic status may be less apparent than in men (Langford et al., 1968).

This section will not attempt exhaustively to review the very rich epidemiological literature. Recent reviews on this topic have been carried out by Guttmann and Benson (1971); Henry and Cassel (1969) and Stamler et al. (1967b). It will try to summarize some of the explanations that may account for the puzzling and often discrepant results obtained in prevalence studies of essential hypertension. These discrepancies have given rise to much discussion about the relative roles of genetic and environmental factors in essential hypertension. Epidemiologists of essential hypertension emphasize the roles of various environmental factors and discount genetic factors.

Because the coefficient of resemblance for blood pressure levels is greater in family members and in spouses, environmental factors must play a major role in the etiology of essential hypertension. But the specific nature of these factors has not been identified. For example, we do not know why blood pressure levels rise with age. If we did know, we might be able to identify the environmental factors that produce the rise. Perhaps, the increase in blood pressure levels with age may be more related to changes in the elasticity of blood vessels.

In any case, and in most populations throughout the world, levels of blood pressure rise with age (Henry and Cassel, 1969; Sokolow and Harris, 1961). Systolic blood pressure levels tend to rise faster with age than diastolic ones. The blood pressure of young persons with blood pressure levels at the upper end of the distribution curve rise faster with age than those with levels in the median range (Harris and Singer, 1968; Julius and Schorck, 1971). In women, the rate of increase of both systolic and diastolic blood pressure is greater than in men in Norway (Bøe et al.; 1957), England (Pickering, 1955, 1961), and the United States (Kagan et al., 1958). In women the increase in blood pressure with age begins earlier (35–40 years) than in men (Platt, 1959; Robinson and Brucer, 1939; Winckelstein and Kantor, 1967). Elevated diastolic levels are less-prevalent in young women and more prevalent in middle-aged ones than in men (Aleksandrow, 1967).

Although the distribution of blood pressure progressively moves toward higher levels and greater variability in levels occurs as people get older, exceptions to these generalizations occur; in some individuals the blood pressure levels remain the same throughout adulthood, whereas in other people they actually decrease with age (Bassett et al., 1966; Stamler et al.; 1958). Increased blood pressure levels in the hypertensive range occur most often in middle life, but they can already be seen in children 5 to 7 years of age (Sokolow and Harris, 1961; Stamler et al., 1958).

The differences in the prevalence of essential hypertension, especially its malignant phase, in black and white Americans remains unexplained. The differences in the course of the disease in men and women have not been accounted for (Perera, 1955; Simpson and Gilchrist, 1958; Smirk, 1957; Sokolow and Perloff, 1961).

THE ROLE OF SOCIOCULTURAL FACTORS IN ESSENTIAL HYPERTENSION AND HIGH BLOOD PRESSURE

Epidemiological studies have not accounted for the difference in the prevalence of essential hypertension in various social and cultural groups. Sociocultural and psychological studies have tentatively identified some of the environmental factors that may play a role in the predisposition and initiation of the disease. These factors may interact with the genetic tendency to the disease. Henry and Cassell (1969) in their exhaustive review have critically examined the evidence for and against the roles of exercise, salt intake, tobacco smoking, malnutrition, illness, obesity, and heredity in essential hypertension. They have concluded that physical exertion, labor, or exercise may be associated with either high or low blood pressure levels. Persons who do not exert themselves may have either high or low levels. Presumably, exertion is associated with high blood pressure only in the predisposed.

Much has been written about the role of salt in essential hypertension. A high salt intake has been associated with very high blood pressure levels in farmers living on the northern isalnd of Japan (Takahashi et al., 1957). Actually, the role of salt in essential hypertension is likely to be an additive one; salt may elevate blood pressure levels only in the presence of preexisting renal damage, caused, for instance, by pyelonephritis (Shapiro, 1963).

A high salt intake may be associated with low blood pressure levels in some cultures and high levels in others. In the United States no relationship has been found between blood pressure levels and the amount of sodium excreted in the urine—an index of salt intake (Dawber et al., 1967). A diet rich in fat is eaten by people with normal blood pressure levels; other people on a lean diet have high blood pressure levels. Other habits, such as smoking tobacco are not associated with high blood pressure levels (Dawber et al., 1967). Malnutrition does not per se reduce the blood pressure or prevent the increase in blood pressure levels with age. Even the traditional view that a strong positive correlation exists between obesity and high blood pressure has been weakened by a careful analysis of the data: Aleksandrow (1967) found that the systolic blood pressure of the obese is 10 to 15 mm Hg higher on the average than that of the underweight. The increased blood pressure in the obese is in part accounted for by the greater volume of the upper arm in the obese. Obese people also have increasing levels of blood pressure with age, but the increase is no faster than in the lean and can, therefore, not be explained on the basis of obesity alone.

Sociocultural factors, other than diet, salt, or obesity play a predisposing or initiating role in essential hypertension (Charvat et al., 1964; Gutmann and Benson, 1971; Henry and Cassel, 1969; Scotch and Geiger, 1963). They are mediated by brain mechanisms (Folkow and Rubinstein, 1966; Henry and Cassel, 1969; Weiner, 1970). When a society is stable, and when its customs, traditions and institutions are well-established and well-structured and its members respond to a predictable sociocultural environment with integrated patterns of psychological adaptation, then blood pressure levels do not become elevated with age. Those who live in a social milieu that is rapidly changing, is unpredictable, dangerous, or unfamiliar—so that psychological adaptation to it is difficult or impossible—tend to develop increasing blood pressure levels with age. Not everyone who lives in such a social milieu develops high blood pressure levels or essential hypertension—probably, only the predisposed do.

Culture change or social chaos may impose adaptive psychological burdens that become intolerable if they also disrupt a person's habitual patterns of psychological adaptation or coping. Patterns of coping are usually established in childhood: if successful, they become habitual. If they become disrupted and are no longer effective, especially during early middle life, blood pressure levels may rise. Some participants in rapid social change and migrants to an urban environment or to another culture are likely to develop high blood pressure levels (Cruz-Coke, 1960; Stamler et al., 1967a; Syme et al., 1964). New roles that have to be assumed in a new setting may be stressful (Scotch, 1961). A change in social or professional status may impose strains on psychological adaptation (Christenson and Hinkle, 1961). Not all persons develop essential hypertension in new settings. Additional factors must play a pathogenetic role. Not everyone is the same in the way he meets and overcomes the challenge of change, migration, a new job, or new relationships in a different setting.

Support for this contention is found in studies on hypertensive women. The relationships of these women to other people are often hostile, combative, and "abrasive." The hypertensive women are less attractive physically. They cannot accept and are resentful of their feminine role. They are careful not to express their angry feelings. They bear secret grudges longer than others. Their marriages are frequently unhappy. Their capacity to be anything but truculent is limited (Harris and Singer, 1968). These women do not

23

adapt well in new social environments. Their truculence only makes it more difficult for them to gain the help and support of others in new settings or when social change occurs. When exposed to danger they fight, or when they are divorced they savor their misfortune.

These psychological and sociocultural factors may play a role in the etiology of essential hypertension but they do not explain in any specific way why black Americans are particularly prone to essential hypertension. Blacks are exposed to similar social changes to those of white Americans. But black Americans have higher blood pressure levels and a higher morbidity and mortality due to hypertensive disease and strokes than their white compatriots. Some blacks are also exposed to more prejudice and violence, especially if poor. In fact, the prevalence of high blood pressure is greater in poor than in middle-class black Americans. Poor black Americans also live in more crowded conditions, have higher rates of divorce, and move more frequently than middle class blacks. They are deeply resentful of police brutality but feel they must keep a rein on expressing their resentments (Harburg et al., 1973).

The correlations between socioeconomic conditions and status and blood pressure levels in black Americans support the hypothesis that sociocultural factors play an etiological role in essential hypertension and hypertensive disease. The data partly elucidate how social and socioeconomic factors may elicit unexpressible or unexpressed anger and resentment in hypertensive parients. In this case the anger is a response to real danger, external prejudice, and violence.

Sociocultural studies are, however, correlational in nature: socioeconomic status, living conditions, and the marital status of patients with different levels of blood pressure are validly related to each other. But the exact nature of the relationships is not clear. The correlations between sociocultural or socioeconomic conditions may or may not be causal to the etiology and pathogenesis of essential hypertension. Such studies should be combined with studies of the social conditons and changes in the lives of patients before or at the time blood pressure levels begin to increase.

THE ROLE OF PSYCHOLOGICAL AND PSYCHOPHYSIOLOGICAL VARIABLES IN ESSENTIAL HYPERTENSION

Relatively few psychiatric studies of the onset conditions of essential hypertension have been carried out. Many obstacles stand in the way of such studies. Very often essential hypertension is discovered on routine examination and it is then impossible to determine when the blood pressure became elevated. Because the level of blood pressure rises with age in many people, individual blood pressure levels should be age-adjusted before they are judged to be normal or not. Generally speaking, this is not done in most studies.

Usually no symptoms accompany early hypertension (Pickering, 1961), although some patients complain of headache, fatigue, weakness, palpitations, loss of appetite, dizziness, true vertigo, and insomnia. They are then found to have elevated blood pressures on routine examination (Ayman, 1930; Ayman and Pratt, 1931; Benedict, 1956; Tucker, 1949, 1950). These symptoms should not be causally ascribed to high blood pressure levels because they are frequently relieved by reassurance, suggestion, or placebos

(Ayman, 1930; Goldring et al., 1956). The symptoms can usually be related to the patient's knowing and being concerned about an elevated blood pressure rather than to the direct effect of the hypertension (Stewart, 1953). In any case, the appearance of these symptoms is not a reliable indication of the onset of essential hypertension. The onset may antedate the symptoms that often occur after the unexpected discovery of the hypertension.

Antecedent and Concomitant Life Events

Relatively prolonged elevations of blood pressure have been reported after man-made disasters (Ruskin et al., 1948) or after prolonged engagement in military combat (Gelshteyn, 1943; Ehrstrom, 1945; Graham, 1945). Not all persons developed high blood pressure under these circumstances, but in those who did, the elevations lasted a maximum of two months and then returned to "normal" levels. The incidence of hypertension in Russia is greater in persons chronically exposed to high levels of noise (Simonson and Brožek, 1959).

The onset of hypertension may occur in the course of everyday events and situations. Similar events may also suddenly alter the course of essential hypertension, so that the disease changes from its benign to its malignant form. Weiss (1942) found that the symptoms of hypertension begin in stressful situations. And Fischer (1961) reported that the onset of hypertension could be correlated in time with the anniversary of an important relative's death. The personal relationship of the patient to the dead relative was "primitive," close, dependent, and ambivalent.

Such formulations about the personal relationships of patients appear and reappear in the psychosomatic literature, not only with respect to patients with hypertension but also with respect to persons who have other diseases or no diseases at all. Despite the lack of apparent specificity of these life events for hypertension, they play a "necessary," if not "sufficient," role in the onset of essential hypertension. Other predisposing factors, including genetic ones, may play additional roles. However, these assertions need be verified with much greater rigor and validated on more than one patient. Reiser and co-workers (1950, 1951a) did so. They found that in 50 percent of 80 patients significant and palpable life events could be identified that preceded or corresponded in time with the known onset of hypertension. Because of the psychological make-up of these patients, the events had particular meanings for their patients.

The psychosocial factors that modify the course of the disease have also been studied by Reiser et al. (1951b). The onset of the malignant phase of primary and secondary hypertension in 12 patients in whom the disease had previously had a benign course was precipitated by interpersonal conflicts about dependency and hostility expressed in sadomasochistic fears. Moreover, these conflicts were very much like those with which the onset of the disease had been correlated. In 76 percent of the patients studied by Chambers and Reiser (1953), the occurrence of cardiac failure in patients with limited cardiac reserve was correlated in time with events that were emotionally significant to the individual patient. Two classes of interpersonal events were identified; those leading to feelings of frustration and rage, and those leading to a feeling of rejection in which the threat of loss of security predominated.

The course of the disease can be improved by the ministrations of a benign and supportive physician combined with the use of drugs (Shapiro and Teng, 1957; Shapiro et al., 1954) or by a thoughtful physician upon whom the patient can depend (Moses et al., 1956; Reiser et al., 1951a; Weiss, 1957).

Such studies—and there are still too few—raise a number of questions about the specific physiological event or events that change the course of the illness. Or is the critical variable that produces the change the "quantity" of the stress rather than any specific event? Or is the change in course a product of the interaction of physiological and psychological factors?

Other Factors: The Role of Salt Intake

The foregoing studies have been repeatedly criticized for being "subjective" and "anecdotal." Pejorative criticism of this kind is easily leveled at clinical studies even when serious attempts are made to verify the reliability of the observation. However, the relative lack of progress in psychosomatic studies of essential hypertension mainly stems from two sources—the impossibility of carrying out predictive studies and a failure to test alternative hypotheses. It may very well be true that inhibited hostility and anger in response to frustration, external danger, and violence may, in some instances, be a necessary condition in the predisposed individual; but it is also possible that this anger does not directly lead to raised blood pressure, but rather leads to changes in diet or in the carrying out of the doctor's instructions once the illness is established, which either further promote hypertension or affect the course of the disease.

One alternative hypothesis to the exclusive etiological role of psychosocial factors is that the individual predisposed to essential hypertension ingests more salt and water than normal people do. Dahl (1958), 1960) and Dahl and Love (1957) have pointed out that there is a linear correlation between the quantity of salt intake and the incidence of essential hypertension. In a cultural group where the intake of salt is low, the probability of some percentage of that group developing essential hypertension is lower than in another group in which there is a greater intake of salt. Cultural factors do seem to play a role in the incidence of hypertension: for example, the illness is unknown in New Guinea, but it is a major cause of death in Japan, where the dietary content of salt is very high. The amount of dietary salt is partly a function of the cultural setting. However, an individual's appetite for salt may be independent of his requirement for it. We are just beginning to learn what accounts for individual variations in salt appetite. For instance, they could be due to altered thresholds in the taste for salt (Fallis et al., 1962; Wotman et al., 1967); however, this has not been confirmed. When 10 patients with essential hypertension were compared with 12 normotensive volunteers, no differences in the detection and recognition thresholds for salt could be discerned. However, when placed on a constant dry diet containing 9 mEq of sodium, the hypertensive patients much preferred to drink water containing 0.15 M sodium chloride than distilled water. They consumed a significantly greater proportion of their total fluid intake as saline and drank more fluids per day. They consumed more than four times as much salt per day as did the volunteers (Schechter et al., 1973). The meaning of this correlation is uncertain. The increased consumption of salt may be related to some aspect of the disease, such as increased serum levels of angiotensin II. However, the preference for salt in some hypertensives may cause high blood pressure levels to be perpetuated. Predictive studies are needed to determine whether individuals predisposed to hypertension show the same salt preference as those who already suffer from it.

Many more studies of this kind will have to be done before conclusions can be reached about the role of a preference for salt in the pathogenesis of essential hypertension. The relationships of feelings and attitudes to salt intake might also be studied, because angry hypertensives may not follow their low-salt diets, may consume more fluids (including alcohol), or may discard their antihypertensive medication when they are disappointed in either their physician or the effectiveness of treatment or are bothered by the side effects of their medications.

Conceptual and Methodological Problems

Psychological studies of patients after the onset of essential hypertension have the implied purpose of uncovering those features of the personality that may play a role in the etiology, pathogenesis, or maintenance of the disease. Since it has not been established that features of the personality studied after disease onset play an etiological or pathogenetic role in essential hypertension (Glock and Lennard, 1957), the logic of this implied research goal is open to question. In order to circumvent this problem, a more careful assertion should be made—that personality factors that characterize hypertensive patients covary with elevated blood pressure levels. Indeed they may; for in the absence of established fact, the hypothesis could be put forward that both the personality features and the elevated blood pressure levels are but the expression of a third variable—for instance, a genetic one or the effect on the brain of some pathophysiological disturbance, such as raised angiotensin levels.

Clinical psychiatric studies of hypertension have suffered from methodological flaws. Many subject variables—such as socioeconomic status, age, and sex—or disease variables—such as the duration and stage of the illness, or whether essential hypertension or some other form is being studied—have often been disregarded. In some studies, blood pressure readings were only taken once. Control subjects have not always been chosen with sufficient care, and in some studies control groups have not been used at all (Crisp, 1963). All findings on one patient population need to be validated on a new population. Most studies are biased because the investigator knows that his patients are hypertensive. Attempts to circumvent this problem have been made. Subjects have been selected for study before they had developed hypertension (Harris et al., 1953; Kalis et al., 1961). Subjects have been chosen because they had a verified family history of hypertension, or because they had a vascular hyperreactivity. As noted previously, not everyone would agree that these subjects are at risk for the development of hypertension. New research strategies are needed: it might be possible to study hypertensive patients before and after they had been rendered normotensive by sinus nerve stimulation (Griffith and Schwartz, 1963; 1964; Schwartz and Griffith, 1967). This method would control for the effects of high blood pressure levels on psychological functioning; and it is preferred because antihypertensive drugs, such as reserpine, have powerful pharmacological effects on the central nervous system and at times produce profound depression. New techniques for

27

studying the personal behavioral and psychological characteristics of hypertensive patients are needed to verify the observations made in the past.

The Central Conflict in Essential Hypertension and Concomitant Personality Patterns

The particular facets of the personality chosen for study at any given time parallel the conceptual trends in vogue at that time in psychiatry. The authors of the early studies of patients with essential hypertension tended to focus on the psychological conflicts of their patients. They concluded that patients with essential hypertension had lifelong and largely unconscious conflicts about the expression of hostility, aggression, resentment, rage, rebellion, ambition or dependency (Alexander, 1939, 1950; Ayman, 1933; Barach, 1928; Binger et al., 1945; Dunbar, 1943; Hambling, 1951, 1952; Harris et al., 1953; Hill, 1935; Miller, 1939; Moschowitz, 1919, Moses et al., 1956; O'Hare, 1920; Palmer, 1950; Saslow et al., 1950; Saul, 1939; Thomas, 1964; Van Der Valk, 1957; Weiss, 1942). The psychological mechanisms used to defend against the emergence of these conflicts led to the development of various personality traits: many patients covered up their anger by an outer friendliness or by exercising self-control (Alexander, 1939; Saul, 1939). Other patients were perfectionistic or had difficulties with those in authority, especially if they rebelled against them (Saslow et al., 1950). The conflicts in some of these patients made them anxious; other patients were depressed.

Binger et al. (1945) agreed that hypertensive patients were angry but stressed that these patients lacked the psychological capacity adequately to integrate, handle, or resolve their conflicts about aggression. Patients were made insecure because they could not be certain that they could handle their anger, external danger, or the fear of separation. Fifty percent of their subjects had lost a parent during childhood; they were sensitized by early experience to separation. In fact, 23 of 24 subjects developed hypertension in a setting of actual or threatened bereavement. It is not particularly surprising then that an important variable in *stabilizing* the course of the disease is a sustained, therapeutic, well-managed relationship with a doctor that undoes the fear of separation (Reiser et al., 1951).

Wolf and Wolff and their associates (1948, 1951, 1953, 1955) studied 103 hypertensive patients and concluded that their latent hostility alerted and prepared them to take offensive action against other people. In contrast with members of a hospital staff, normotensive patients, and patients who suffered from bronchial asthma and vasomotor rhinitis, many of the hypertensive patients preferred offensive action to thoughtful reflection. They were tense, suspicious, and wary. Others tried to please and placate those that they feared, rather than take offensive action against them. Hypertensive patients who were prepared to fight were often outwardly calm, easy-going, and restrained.

All of these studies have been criticized because they are based on subjective impression (Davies, 1971): many critics are dissatisfied with the methods of clinical observation and inference. Yet it is remarkable how consistent the clinical descriptions of hypertensive patients are. Nonetheless, they should be verified by psychological tests, such as those of Saslow and his co-workers (1950). They confirmed the fact that hypertensive patients had certain traits; they were less overtly assertive and manifested compulsive character traits more often than normotensive patients who had personality disorders. Wolf and Wolff's studies emphasized that the latent hostility of hypertensive patients was directed at other people, but it was hidden from them by various traits. Thaler and her co-workers (1957) and Weiner and his (1962) further attempted to specify the nature of the hypertensive patient's interpersonal relationships by studying how these patients perceive and interact with their physicians. The implicit aim of these studies was to identify how hypertensive patients perceive other people and how that perception affects their relationships to them. These studies made no explicit or implicit assumption that either the patient's perception of or relationships with others had etiologic or pathogenetic significance for the disease. They found that hypertensive subjects perceive other people as dangerous, derisive, and untrustworthy. Because of this perception, patients attempt to maintain a distant relationship. Paradoxically, they provoke others and are alert to anger and hostility—the very reactions they most fear.

When hypertensive patients successively maintained their distance and avoided relationships, the blood pressure levels remain unchanged, but when this habitual defensive style fails, *critical* elevations of blood pressure occur.

This interpersonal style in the manner with which hypertensive subjects defend against personal involvements was also described by Grace and Graham (1952) who verified their findings in a later study (Graham et al., 1962b). The characteristic attitude of hypertensive patients consists of an "awareness of threat of bodily harm, without any possibility of running away or fighting back." Implicit in this description was an inhibited desire to fight danger.

The observations of Thaler and co-workers (1957) were put to the test by Sapira and co-workers (1971) by a different method: 19 hypertensive and 15 normotensive patients were shown two movies, one depicted a rude and disinterested physician and the other a physician who was at ease and related with patients in a warm and kindly manner. The hypertensive patients had significantly greater blood pressure and heart rate responses while viewing the two films and during a later interview. The hypertensive patients denied perceiving any differences between the actions and attitudes of the two physicians. The normotensive group could tell the difference in the behavior of the two physicians. The interviewer evoked greater blood pressure response in hypertensive patients when he played the roles of the physician in the movies than when he did not (Sapira et al., 1971). The authors postulate that the hypertensive patients screen out the perception of the differences between the "good" and "bad" doctor while still showing blood pressure responses in order to defend against their cardiovascular hyperreactivity. The patients in this study did not state that they could tell the difference between a "good" and "bad" doctor because to admit that they saw one would be tantamount to seeing the other.

If hypertensive patients avoid the perception of potentially hostile and dangerous relationships they should differ from patients in whom high blood pressure levels are the consequence of kidney disease; but they do not. Ostfeld and Lebovitz (1959) studied 50 patients with essential hypertension and compared them to 50 with renovascular hypertension. They concluded on the basis of MMPI and Rorschach test findings that no psychological differences existed between the two groups. Patients in both groups reacted similarly to anxiety by equivalent elevations of blood pressure. The authors concluded, therefore, that no particular psychological factors play any etiological role in essential hypertension. Their observations suggest that once high blood pressure is established, anxiety may further raise it. Anxiety, regardless of its source, may sustain or further elevate preexisting blood pressure levels, regardless of etiology. Because of this study, the contribution of psychological factors to the etiology and pathogenesis is questionable. In particular, the role that anger, rage, or hostility plays in inciting the disease remains enigmatic.

In an attempt to verify the role of anger or hostility in the production of high blood pressure levels, psychotic persons have been studied. Psychotic persons are often either overtly angry, hostile, and suspicious, or they struggle against the direct expression of such feelings. Miller (1939) tested this hypothesis. He found much higher blood pressure levels in patients who had hostile, paranoid delusions or who were agitated and depressed than in patients who had grandiose delusions or who were depressed and apathetic. But Monroe and co-workers (1961) could not verify Miller's findings on 766 hospitalized psychotic patients.

This research strategy is probably not a good one. Neither study takes into account the expected prevalence of high blood pressure in a population of this age group. Psychotic people also vary a great deal, and psychiatrists cannot agree among themselves about their diagnosis. Therefore, two populations of psychotic persons are not comparable if different psychiatrists make the diagnoses. Finally, these studies are based on the belief that overt or unexpressed anger alone produces high blood pressure.

Because no agreement has been reached about the role of hostility in the etiology or pathogenesis of essential hypertension, it might be worthwhile to review the attempts to verify clinical impressions by predictive psychiatric and psychological studies. Notable among these are studies carried out by Alexander and his colleagues (1968). The psychological criteria used to diagnose hypertensive patients in this study were that they were

> struggling against aggressive feelings and had difficulties in asserting them. The patients were afraid to lose the affection of others and had to control the expression of their hostility. In childhood the patients were prone to outbursts of rage and aggression. As they matured and developed the angry attacks came under control. Consequently they became overtly compliant and unassertive. As adults they perservered doggedly, often against insuperable obstacles. When promoted to executive positions they encountered difficulties because they could not assert themselves or make others follow their orders. They were overconscientious and too responsible. Their conscientiousness only increased their feelings of resentment at self-imposed tasks.
>
> ALEXANDER, 1968

The onset of hypertension was brought about by events that mobilized hostility and the urge for self-assertion but at the same time prohibited their free expression.

About 40 percent of the hypertensive patients were correctly diagnosed by nine judges. Male hypertensive patients were more-often correctly diagnosed than female ones. This study attests to the fact that these criteria may not be correct in all patients, especially not women. It suggests that patients with essential hypertension are psychologically heterogeneous. The psychological heterogeneity of hypertensive patients may reflect the physiological heterogeneity and stage of the disease. Alexander's study was an attempt to validate his formulations about aggressive conflicts and how they are expressed. A better research strategy is to predict before onset who will develop essential hypertension. But, as has been noted, no criteria for predicting who is at risk for the disease have been developed, except that it occurs more frequently in the children of parents with hypertension.

Thomas (1957, 1958, 1961, 1964a, 1967) and her co-workers (Bruce and Thomas, 1953; Thomas et al., 1964a, b; Thomas and Ross, 1963) carried out such a prospective study. They administered psychological tests to 1,200 medical students and their parents in 1953. By 1967, 400 parents had died. Of these, 100 had died of the complications of hypertensive or coronary artery disease. No striking definitive psychological differences were found between the offspring of parents dying of hypertension and heart disease and the offspring of parents dead of other diseases, or those still alive and well. However, the children of hypertensive parents tended to be more aggressive and hostile and to feel more inadequate. They had compulsive character traits. Although no huge differences were uncovered between the offspring of hypertensive parents and the offspring of those who were not hypertensive, these studies tend to confirm the observations obtained by retrospective studies.

Clinical psychiatric impressions have also partly been verified by the use of psychological tests after the onset of hypertension. Many of these studies are hard to compare, as the tests employed differ and the medical data on the patients are not described. Often it is not clear how frequently blood pressure was taken, whether the level had been elevated for days, months, or years, or whether it was affected by the manner in which it was taken (Ostfeld and Shekelle, 1967). The question of whether the patient had essential or some other form of hypertension is usually left unanswered. In fact, patients at risk for related diseases are similar psychologically to patients with essential hypertension.

Patients at risk for or with coronary heart disease are like patients with essential hypertension (Friedman and Rosenman, 1959; Jenkins et al., 1967; Rosenman, 1969; Rosenman and Friedman, 1963; Rosenman et al., 1964, 1966). Many factors predispose to coronary artery disease but high blood pressure is certainly one of them. In studies that were both retrospective and predictive, a behavior pattern has been described that is prognostic of coronary artery disease. The patients are "driven," ambitious, and aggressive, and pressure themselves to be productive and to meet deadlines. They are competitive, restless in manner, and staccato in speech; they hurry constantly and have an enhanced sense of the urgency of time. The risk of coronary artery disease is heightened when this style is associated with elevated blood pressure and serum lipoprotein levels (Rosenman and Friedman, 1963). In the hands of other investigators the results have not been as clear-cut (Friedman et al., 1968), perhaps because socioeconomic, cultural, and other environmental variables also influence the behavior pattern (Keith et al., 1965). The description of this behavior pattern is reminiscent of the behavior pattern of women with borderline hypertension (Harris et al., 1953; Kalis et al., 1961; Harris and Singer, 1968).

Male patients with borderline blood pressure elevations seem more "nervous and excitable" than matched comparison subjects. They are submissive, lethargic, introverted, lacking in self-confidence, sensitive and suspicious, and derive no pleasure from sexual relationships (Hamilton, 1942; Harburg et al., 1964). Patients with borderline hypertension do not constitute a uniform subgroup. Some young men with this stage or form of essential hypertension have a high cardiac output; other borderline hypertensives have a normal cardiac output.

Attempts to relate blood pressure levels to various features of the personality have also been made. Brower (1947a, b) discovered a negative correlation between diastolic blood pressure levels and good social adjustment, and a positive correlation with depressive, psychopathic, and hypochondriacal scores on the MMPI.

Cattell and Scheier (1959) demonstrated a positive relationship between systolic blood pressure levels, exuberance, and optimism about attaining long-range goals. But the hypertensive patients also lacked confidence in their ability to perform in novel situations.

A number of other psychological studies have found no differences between patients with other diseases or with different forms of high blood pressure: when four groups, each consisting of 15 patients with duodenal ulcer, essential hypertension, neuromuscular tension, and control subjects were compared, the patients in the three clinical groups scored higher than the control group on scales of depression, hysteria, psychopathy, and hypochrondriasis (Innes et al., 1959; Lewinsohn, 1956; Robinson, 1962; Storment, 1951).

Patients who do not have borderline hypertension but who do have higher blood pressure levels have been described as insecure and submissive, yet sensitive to criticism about their anger. A test of this observation was made by criticizing hypertensive patients and normotensive subjects while they responded to the Thematic Apperception Test. Twelve normotensive and only one hypertensive refused to continue with the test. Both groups became less verbally aggressive when criticized (Matarazzo, 1954). Neiberg (1957) concluded that neither patients nor control subjects inhibited their anger when criticized.

Ostfeld and Lebovitz (1959, 1960) found no significant psychological differences between patients with essential or renovascular hypertension and normotensive subjects. The patients did show increases in blood pressure greater than those of normotensive subjects during a discussion of distressing life experiences or interviews. The patients and subjects who were most emotionally labile were also likely to show the greatest changes in blood pressure levels.

Psychological tests can reveal whether patients are anxious or more emotionally labile. Some psychoneurotic patients are both. A number of studies have compared hypertensive and psychoneurotic patients with each other and with supposedly normal subjects. There are many psychological similarities between patients, but they differ equally from normals. On the other hand, the most neurotic patients do not have the highest blood pressure levels (Robinson, 1962, 1964; Sainsbury, 1960, 1964).

The most sophisticated study to date related the psychological features of patients to various measures of the circulation. By the use of the proper controls, hypertensive patients were found to be more emotional, tense, unstable and excitable, guilt-ridden, timid, insecure and sexually inhibited than normotensive patients. They were deferential to others and abased themselves. The more deferential they were, the greater the peripheral resistance and resting blood pressure levels. The more they abased themselves, the higher the resting blood pressure levels. The more they were emotionally stimulated, the greater were the changes in diastolic and systolic blood pressure levels. Those hypertensive patients who expressed interest in members of the opposite sex had high heart rates and diastolic blood pressure levels. The more anxious and tense they were, the higher the basal peripheral resistance, and the more it increased on stimulation (Pilowsky et al., 1973).

The tentative conclusion can be reached that the clinical psychiatric traits and psychological states occur in some, but not in all, hypertensive patients. There is psychological heterogeneity. On the other hand, a relationship exists between emotionality, excessive vascular hyperreactivity, and blood pressure variability in patients with essential and renovascular hypertension.

Essential hypertension runs in families—a fact that is not well-understood, but that is quoted in support of genetic factors in the disease. The family aggregation of essential hypertension could also be understood in terms of altered family relationships. If hypertensive parents perceive the human environment, including their children, as hostile and dangerous, they could intimidate their children.

Few studies of the families of hypertensive patients have been conducted. Harburg and co-workers (1965) found that patients with the most labile blood pressure did not like their fathers because they were domineering, stern, and socially ambitious for their families. Davies (1970) found that blood pressure variability and levels had to be treated separately when they were correlated with parental attitudes. Subjects with high basal blood pressure levels reported that their fathers were tolerant. Patients with lower levels were more critical of their fathers. In this connection it should be recalled that hypertensive patients when they are compensated psychologically tend to eschew criticizing other people (Sapira et al., 1971). Saul (1939) was one of the few ever to study the mothers of hypertensive patients. He ascribed the patients' repressed feelings of hostility to the domineering behavior of their mothers.

We still lack the kinds of detailed studies of families of hypertensive patients that have been done on the families of patients with bronchial asthma, ulcerative colitis, or rheumatoid arthritis. We also know rather little about the psychological make-up of patients in childhood, or how they are treated by their parents to predispose them to essential hypertension.

Reiser (1970) postulated that in infancy these children may cry a lot. During crying, the child expires against a partially closed glottis and increases intrathoracic pressure, diminishing the venous return to the heart and the cardiac output. The peripheral resistance and heart rate rise as a consequence. The Valsalva maneuver, carried out in adulthood, mimics the changes brought about by crying. In hypertensive patients the maneuver produces more than the usual increase in blood pressure. Reiser's suggestion has not been put to the test. He implies that the crying is the child's response to inadequate or inappropriate mothering. As a result of repeated bouts of crying the circulation becomes "conditioned" to respond with excessive blood pressure responses. It becomes hyperreactive to stimuli, including emotional ones. But we do not know whether babies who cry excessively or repeatedly are at risk for essential hypertension. Perhaps some are, because they are born with a hyperreactive cardiovascular system. The hyperreactivity may be genotypic, but the crying is provoked by the mother who does not satisfy the child, eliciting the hypertensive phenotype. To complicate the matter further, children vary temperamentally at birth. Some are easily satisfied, others are not: the mother should not receive the blame for being the only cause of the child's unhappiness.

Studies should be done of the families of hypertensive patients and of the psychological development of children of hypertensive patients as well as of children with elevated blood pressure levels.

Studies of the Psychophysiological Correlates
of Blood Pressure and of Essential Hypertension in Man

Psychophysiological studies on patients with essential hypertension have been carried out with several purposes in mind: (1) to determine whether persons who later develop essential hypertension can be identified in advance; (2) to assess the role of simple and complex psychological stimuli and the emotions they elicit in changing blood pressure; and (3) to determine whether there are differences in cardiovascular dynamics between hypertensive and normotensive subjects. For example, hypnotic trances have been induced to study changes in blood pressure, and meditative states and biofeedback techniques have been used to lower the blood pressure of hypertensive patients and normal subjects.

Psychophysiological studies are fraught with technical, methodological, and conceptual problems. The fact that elevations of blood pressure occur in hypertensive patients in response to psychological stimuli does not constitute prima facie evidence that psychological stimuli have etiologic or pathogenetic relevance to the disease. Short-term changes in blood pressure produced in the laboratory do not necessarily provide us with important insights into the nature of sustained high blood pressure, diastolic and systolic. A major methodological problem in such studies is the fact that—with the exception of Brod's important studies—there has been a tendency to study one or two cardiovascular variables, such as the heart rate and blood pressure. Studies that use only two parameters of cardiovascular function may be misleading, because profound hemodynamic changes (for example, in regional blood flow) may occur without a discernible change in blood pressure. Several cardiovascular variables must be studied simultaneously in psychophysiological studies.

Because of the repeated clinical observation that patients with essential hypertension harbor strong feelings of anger, there have been attempts to correlate anger with cardiovascular responses (Moses et al., 1956; Schachter, 1957) and to contrast these responses to those obtained when fear, pain or anxiety are elicited. Pain can be produced by immersion of the patient's hand in ice water at 3° C for one minute, anger is stimulated by insulting and abusing the subject, and fear can be produced by a mild electric shock (Ax, 1953).

In the hypertensive patients greater increments in blood pressure occurred in the three situations designed to produce, respectively, fear, pain, and anger (Schachter, 1957). In both the pain and anger conditions, diastolic blood pressure rose significantly because of an increased peripheral resistance, whereas fear produced increases in systolic blood pressure as the cardiac output increased.

In Schachter's (1957) experiment, the situation designed to produce pain is also

34

conducive to vasoconstriction; immersion of a limb in ice water has often been used to measure blood pressure reactivity in normal and hypertensive subjects. The effects of mild pain and vasoconstriction are confounded in this experiment. Pain and other feelings interact with vasoconstriction; blood pressure reactivity is greater if the cold immersion test is given to anxious patients (White and Gildea, 1937). The blood pressure reactivity is also greater in neurotic (Malmo and Shagass, 1952) and angry patients than in calm ones (Cranston et al., 1949). Heart rate and blood pressure changes have been used to infer (Schachter, 1957) or measure the associated humoral changes that correlate with specific affects. When aggression and active emotional states are elicited in subjects, norepinephrine secretion occurs. Whereas when anger is handled intrapunitively, urinary epinephrine levels are increased in normal subjects (Cohen et al., 1957; Cohen and Silverman, 1959; Elmadjian et al., 1957). The relationship between the blood pressure, catecholamine excretion, and mental stress depends in part on the state and stage of hypertension. It may be that borderline cases or young male hypertensive patients have different cardiovascular dynamics with different excretion levels of the catecholamines than do patients with well-established hypertension or normals. Nestel (1969) has reexamined this problem by studying 17 normotensive subjects and 20 hypertensive patients with a mean resting blood pressure of 147/95 mm Hg. Basal urinary excretion levels of norepinephrine and epinephrine were the same in both groups of subjects. The subjects were asked to solve visual puzzles—the Raven's matrix test—for 40 minutes. Much greater increments in systolic ($\Delta = 35$ mm Hg) and diastolic ($\Delta = 25$ mm Hg) blood pressure occurred in the labile hypertensive group than in the normotensive group. The urinary output of norepinephrine and epinephrine rose in all subjects but the increases were significantly greater in the hypertensive patients, rising in 17 of the 20. By comparison, the urinary output of the neurotransmitters rose in only 7 of the 17 normotensive subjects. Mean postexperimental levels of both catecholamines were also higher in the former group. The changes in urinary catecholamine levels correlated significantly with changes in blood pressure levels, particularly in the labile hypertensive group.

Apparently patients with labile hypertension respond to a complex psychological task by increased sympathetic nervous activity and greater blood pressure responses. More direct approaches to the evaluation of sympathetic activity in this group of patients have also been made. Attempts to evaluate overall sympathetic activity in patients with labile hypertension by estimating dopamine β-hydroxylase (DBH) levels have not been successful. No individual differences in levels occur and there is no relationship between DBH levels, the blood pressure levels, or the age of subjects. DBH levels are lower in black than in white persons and in men than in women. The reduction of the blood pressure by drugs in borderline or labile hypertensive patients does not reduce serum DBH activity (Horwitz et al., 1973).

Whether discernible differences in physiological responses occur in different affective states continues to be a moot point (Buss, 1961). Harris and his co-workers (1965) do not believe in such differences. They performed cardiac catheterization and serial blood-chemical studies while intense, lifelike fear and anger were induced under hypnosis. Similar physiological responses accompanied fear and anger. Fear and angry responses were both associated with a 33 percent increase in cardiac index, with a 50 percent rise in the heart rate, a 20 percent fall in stroke volume, a 10 mm Hg increase in blood pressure, and a 13 percent fall in peripheral resistance. The respiratory rate doubled and six subjects developed a respiratory alkalosis. Mean levels of plasma hydrocortisone and plasma nonesterified fatty acids doubled. A β-adrenergic blocking agent reduced the cardioaccelerator response due to fear but not due to anger. The agent failed to block the increases of cardiac output, plasma hydrocortisone, and free fatty acids. In three subjects the entire experiment was repeated several weeks later and the results were replicated. Therefore, under hypnosis it is impossible to discriminate between the physiological correlates of fear and anger in normal subjects. In other experiments, anger produces qualitatively similar but quantitatively greater cardiovascular responses. Hokanson (1961a, b) harassed subjects while they were counting. He found that the more hostile subjects had brisker increases in systolic and diastolic blood pressure. Those who expressed their anger and hostility openly had a great fall in systolic blood pressure when the experiment was over, which suggested, Hokanson argued, that the failure to express these feelings, due to guilt or anxiety, delayed the fall in blood pressure to preexperimental levels. Graham et al. (1960, 1962a) hypnotized two groups of normal subjects. A psychological attitude correlated with hives was suggested to one group, and an attitude of unexpressible rage to another group. Significant skin temperature changes occurred when hives were suggested, and increases in diastolic blood pressure when rage was suggested. Inhibited or partially expressed hostile verbal content in awake subjects can be evaluated by the method of Gottschalk and Hambidge (1955) while blood pressure is measured. Using this technique, Kaplan et al. (1960) found that while hypertensive subjects spoke, their blood pressures rose. In contrast, while normotensive subjects spoke, their blood pressures fell. In hypertensive subjects a significant relationship was found between the intensity of the hostile content of speech and the diastolic blood pressure levels.

In normal subjects the evidence that different feelings, such as fear or anger, are correlated with specific cardiovascular or humoral responses is by no means established. In some studies specific physiological responses to specific feelings have been demonstrated in normal subjects. In other studies, the degree but not the specific kind of physiological response is related to anger that is partially inhibited in its expression. Psychophysiological studies in normal subjects may be relevant to the etiology of high blood pressure, but they do not prove that anger or hostility specifically raise the blood pressure any more than fear does. Responses to feelings in normal subjects are often different in degree, duration, or kind than in hypertensive subjects.

Many studies have been designed to show that psychological stimuli of various kinds in the laboratory do elicit changes in blood pressure in hypertensive subjects, and that these changes were greater or longer-lasting than in normal subjects (Jost et al., 1952).

Wolf and Wolff (1951) interviewed 203 normotiensive subjects and 103 subjects with blood pressure levels of 160/95 mm Hg or more. Although the hypertensive subjects were usually affable and friendly to the experimenter, their blood pressure rose more during the interview. It did not do so consistently, however, because different changes in cardiovascular dynamics occurred with different feelings. When the predominant feeling in the interview was restrained hostility or anxiety, the cardiac output did not change, but the peripheral resistance rose. With overt anxiety, the cardiac output increased and the peripheral resistance fell. With feelings of despair and of being overwhelmed, both cardiac output and peripheral resistance fell. An association between specific feelings and specific changes in the circulation has not always been observed. Changes in blood pressure do occur during interviews; but the changes may have more to do with the speed with which the subject talks than with the feelings he expresses. Nonetheless, hypertensive patients differ from normotensive ones—even when they talk with the same speed, their blood pressure responses last longer, even after they fall silent (Innes et al., 1959). Innes also found that some neurotic and some hypertensive patients share a common psychological characteristic that he called "emotional lability" (Davies, 1971).

Whether specific emotions produce specific alterations of cardiovascular function has not been settled. Studies in animals support the view that specific emotions are associated with specific cardiovascular responses; studies in humans tend not to (Cannon, 1929). Both Lacey and his co-workers (1952, 1953, 1958) and Wenger and his (1961) have pointed out that changes in cardiovascular function occur against a background of different and individual resting levels and fluctuations in the baseline of heart rate, blood pressure, and peripheral resistance. Although intraindividual autonomically mediated response patterns to psychological stimuli, feelings, and emotional states may be fairly consistent, marked differences between patterns occur when two subjects are compared. Some individuals respond with a particular pattern of cardiovascular responses regardless of the stimulus used. The individual response specificity to various stimuli has also been observed in hypertensive patients (Engel and Bickford, 1961): they responded to various stimuli (such as lights, sounds, mental arithmetic, exercise, and the cold-pressor test) by increases in systolic blood pressure and not by other cardiovascular responses. Their systolic blood pressure responses were greater than in normal subjects and did not depend on the stimulus used. The magnitude of these responses was always greater than in normal subjects. Larger responses are elicited by psychological stimuli as well as physical stimuli such as sounds and immersing the hand in cold water (Reiser et al., 1951a). The blood pressure responses to cold may last for several days.

Pfeiffer and Wolf (1950) used the stress interview to study the renal circulation in 23 hypertensive and 13 normotensive subjects. The renal blood flow fell and the filtration fraction increased in both groups. Presumably, these changes were due to constriction of the renal glomerular arterioles, and they could be conducive to the release of renin. It may well be that such renal changes with psychological stimuli are important in hypertensive subjects; but some additional factors must be involved in the pathogenesis of hypertension, because both groups showed the same changes in renal function. Stressful interviews that had personal significance to hypertensive patients reduced renal blood flow (Wolf et al., 1948) and elicited brisk pressor responses—a rise of 14 mm Hg (Wolf et al., 1955)—and even greater mean blood pressure responses (26.5 mm Hg) in another study (Hardyck and Singer, 1962).

But blood pressure changes in normotensive subjects and hypertensive patients are not only produced by feelings; intellectual tasks and pain also elicit brisk responses. Brod et al. (1959, 1960, 1962, 1970) used mental arithmetic performed under duress to produce increases in arterial blood pressure, muscle blood flow, splanchnic vasoconstriction, and cardiac output in normotensive and hypertensive subjects. More renal vasoconstriction and less vasodilation in muscle was found in hypertensive subjects. The hemodynamic changes and elevations of blood pressure persisted longer in the hypertensive subjects than in the normotensive group. These results must be evaluated bearing in mind that six of the eight normotensive subjects, but only two of the ten hypertensive subjects, were women. Sex differences in cardiovascular reactivity are known to occur. The *patterns* of physiological change Brod has demonstrated in human subjects have also been produced in animals by brain stimulation. The pathways in the brain that regulate this pattern of change are known (Folkow and Rubinstein, 1966; Löfving, 1961; Uvnäs, 1960).

With simple painful stimuli, hypertensive and normotensive subjects with a family history of hypertension have more-rapid and brisker blood pressure responses than normal subjects have. No significant changes in peripheral resistance occur in hypertensive patients with pain. Subjects with a family history of hypertension increase their cardiac output and, therefore, their blood pressure (Shapiro, 1960a, b). The degree and duration of the blood pressure responses to various stimuli and tasks are greater in hypertensive patients than in normal subjects. This increased responsivity occurs both in essential and renovascular hypertension (Ostfeld and Lebovitz, 1959, 1960). In patients with essential hypertension and renovascular hypertension, anxiety produces similar elevations of blood pressure that last equally long. The similar blood pressure responses in different forms of hypertension have been interpreted to mean that psychological factors played no etiological role in essential hypertension. Alternative interpretations are possible: anxiety may interact with some mechanism common to both forms of hypertension to raise the blood pressure. Although anxiety may not play an etiological role, it may help to sustain both forms of hypertension by repeatedly raising blood pressure further. Psychophysiological studies must compare patients with different forms of hypertension like Ostfeld and Lebovitz (1959) did, and take into account the stage and state of the different forms of the disease. It has been suggested that although renal factors may play a prepotent role early in essential hypertension, they are later supplanted by sustaining neurogenic mechanisms. The reverse sequence has also been suggested.

Whatever the sequence may be, psychological factors may be mediated by one set of physiological mechanisms at one stage of the disease and by another set at another stage to raise the blood pressure.

Psychophysiological studies have shown that each person responds physiologically to many different stimuli in his own manner; hypertensive persons also have larger blood pressure responses. Subjects in the psychophysiological laboratory also respond psychologically in their own particular ways. In most studies, the experimenter has attempted to provoke a particular feeling in his subject. In more recent studies, feelings were not provoked. Instead, the experimenter or an observer of the interaction of the experimenter and the subject watched the individual psychological style of the subject. Innes and his colleagues (1959) showed that the speed with which a subject talks is individual and is related to his blood pressure responses.

In other experiments, observations were focused on the style in which the subject and experimenter related to each other, while the blood pressure and other hemodynamic changes were measured. Weiner et al. (1962) found that hypertensive subjects were more unreactive physiologically than normotensive ones, because they interacted little with the experimenter. One hypertensive subject who had previously been unresponsive physiologically was persuaded against his will to undergo the laboratory procedure on a second occasion. He equated the second experiment with a threat to his life, his distant style crumbled, and a very brisk, long-lasting blood pressure response occurred. These experiments demonstrate that the nature of the experimenter-subject relationship, and the effectiveness of a habitual style of relating to the experimenter may be the critical determinants in producing cardiovascular changes in the laboratory. As long as a style "works" no changes occur in normotensive or hypertensive subjects. The detailed findings of this study have been verified (McKegney and Williams, 1967; Williams and McKegney, 1965; Williams et al., 1972a). The findings shed some light on the complex interactions between the nature of the subject-experimenter relationship, the manner in and success with which subjects cope with a task and an experimenter, and changes in cardiovascular function.

Hypertensive patients have individual styles of relating to physicians and experimenters in the laboratory. They keep their distance from them and avoid close personal involvements. They eschew relationships because they perceive the physician as hostile, dangerous, coercive, or ungiving. If they cannot avoid the relationship, their blood pressure responses are brisker and more prolonged than those of normotensive patients (Shapiro, 1973; Thaler et al., 1957; Weiner et al., 1962).

"Coping" and "defensive" styles in man may be the critical intervening variables between the perception of a psychosocial stimulus, the psychological response (including the emotional one) to that perception, and the individual physiological response to the stimulus. If these styles are successful, little physiological change occurs. If not successful, changes do occur. The changes are greater and last longer in hypertensive patients than in normotensive ones. The specific feelings that a stimulus provokes are not associated with specific physiological changes. Anger does not uniquely raise the blood pressure. Other feelings, such as fear and pain, also do. Rather each person responds physiologically in his own manner to a variety of feelings and stimuli. Hypertensive patients respond with brisker blood pressure responses that last longer to a variety of psychological tasks and feelings, as well as to cold and pain. Their cardiovascular responses are predetermined, individual, and hyperreactive for unknown reasons. Their responses may reflect an intrinsic defect in the regulation of blood pressure that may antedate the disease. Hypertensive patients also have individual psychological responses to the experimenter and laboratory and cope differently with pain, cold, and cognitive tasks.

Studies on the Conditioning of Cardiovascular Responses in Man

Psychophysiological experiments on hypertensive patients in the laboratory are complex and difficult to control. Multiple variables such as the nature of the subject-experimenter interaction, the psychological responses to pain or various tasks, and the effect of medication are not easily quantified or controllable. Therefore, a number of investigators have preferred to use various forms of conditioning procedures that are much more easily controlled to elicit blood pressure and other cardiovascular responses.

Human subjects have been conditioned by classical and operant techniques while direct or indirect measurements of blood flow in the extremities, heart rate, or blood pressure are made (Zeaman and Smith, 1965). Classical conditioning stimuli produce vasoconstriction in the extremities. Once a conditioned response (CR) in man has been established, the conditioning stimulus may generalize to the experimenter or the whole laboratory and the CR is set off (Bykov, 1947). The CRs are associated with changes in the caliber of blood vessels in the skin of the extremities. But because blood flow in the splanchnic bed is much more difficult to measure in intact human beings, we do not know directly whether changes in splanchnic flow that are directly relevant to increases in blood pressure can also be conditioned. We can only infer changes in splanchnic blood flow from other studies that show that vascular changes in the skin are usually the reciprocal of those occurring in the splanchnic bed.

Nonetheless, studies on conditioned vasoconstriction in the extremities and increases in blood pressure have heuristic values for hypertension research. Conditioned vasoconstriction in human subjects can be produced not only by simple conditioning stimuli, such as a tone, but also by tasks, such as mental arithmetic (Abramson, 1944: Abramson and Ferris, 1940; Figar, 1965; Petyelina, 1952; Tomaszewski, 1937), or by words. Words related to simple conditioning stimuli tend to produce even brisker skin and blood pressure responses than the simple stimuli themselves (Bykov, 1947). When conflicting stimuli are used, the largest blood pressure responses occur. Sleep abolishes conditioned vasoconstriction. When the patient is awake, awareness of, and attention to the stimulus determine the speed of the establishment of a conditioned vasoconstrictor response (Lacey, 1950; Lacey and Smith, 1954).

Conditioned cardiovascular responses have been established and compared in normotensive and hypertensive subjects. In human subjects in the early stages of essential hypertension, peripheral vasoconstrictor responses are brisker and extinguish less readily than in normotensive subjects (Figar, 1965; Kaminskiy, 1951; Miasnikov, 1954). As the disease progresses, the conditioned responses decrease progressively, presumably because vasoconstriction is already intense. It is difficult, however, to assess these studies because the patients used in these studies were not well-classified: they may have had essential or some other form of hypertension. These studies suggest, nonetheless, that early in the disease vascular hyperreactivity is greater and lasts longer (Page, 1960).

Small but statistically significant and reliable *decreases* in systolic and diastolic blood pressure have been obtained by operant conditioning techniques in normotensive (e.g., Shapiro et al., 1969, 1970) and in hypertensive subjects. The changes in systolic blood pressure obtained by operant means in five of seven hypertensive subjects is of the order of 16 to 34 mm Hg (Benson et al., 1971). The fall in blood pressure is probably not permanent, so that one cannot as yet ascertain whether operant procedures have a role in the treatment of human hypertension.

The studies have been met with some criticism (Blanchard and Young, 1973). As in all psychophysiological experiments, a number of uncontrollable variables occur: they include the subject's knowledge of the experimenter's intentions to lower blood pressure, the effect instructions have on the subject, and the subject's relationship to the experimenter—all of which influence the results. Unless these variables are controlled, the assertion cannot be made that operant or biofeedback procedures lower the blood pressure. In fact, the blood pressure of hypertensive patients can be made to rise and fall when subjects are forcefully instructed to raise or lower their blood pressure. Significant changes in blood pressure also occur with progressive muscular relaxation, but only when the physician encourages the patient to relax. The direction and degree of change in blood pressure equal those obtained by biofeedback techniques that include both instruction and relaxation (Redmond et al., 1974).

40

Psychophysiological Studies of Blood Pressure in a Naturalistic Setting

Much has been learned about the correlations between psychological and physiological variables from laboratory and conditioning studies. Variations in blood pressure could not be studied over the long term and in everyday settings until a method had been developed that would continuously measure the blood pressure. With this nonintrusive method, it becomes possible to relate changes in blood pressure to daily events and the psychological responses that they occasion. Sokolow and his co-workers (1970) studied 124 hypertensive patients in this manner. Marked variations in blood pressure occurred depending on the changing events of the day. For example, one middle-aged student had a blood pressure of 160/95 mm Hg while anticipating a campus interview, and 100/82 mm Hg while at home talking to her son.

An analysis of the changes in 50 hypertensive patients lead to the conclusion that the highest systolic blood pressure levels and pulse rates occur when patients are alert, anxious, or under pressure. The highest diastolic blood pressure levels occur when the patients are anxious or pressured. Contentment lowers levels. Sokolow and his co-workers (1970) also found that the most anxious, hostile, and depressed patients were the ones most likely to develop hypertensive disease and all its complications. This finding should not be surprising, as these patients also had the highest blood pressure levels.

These studies relate high blood pressure levels to the emotional state of patients. They should be viewed with caution. Blood pressure levels vary with behavioral as well as emotional states. They are low in sleep and increase markedly on awakening. Acute increases occur with pain or during coitus. Blood pressure levels are not a stable function—they are subject to circadian rhythms upon which pain, excitement, mental work, anxiety, and anger are superimposed.

ANIMAL MODELS OF ESSENTIAL HYPERTENSION

High Blood Pressure Produced by Conditioning Techniques

The study of animals with high blood pressure has alerted us to the complexity of the various factors that predispose, initiate, and sustain high blood pressure. They have significantly contributed to the elucidation of the mechanisms involved. The techniques used to produce blood pressure elevations in animals vary from constricting the renal artery to exposing animals to "white" noise. In this section, particular attention will be paid to the results obtained by the use of conditioning techniques.

The conditioning procedures take many different forms: unconditioned stimuli (Us), classical and avoidance procedures, and the production of an experimental neurosis have been used to produce elevations of blood pressure (Anderson and Brady, 1971, 1973; Beier, 1940; Bykov, 1947; Forsyth, 1968; 1969; Gantt, 1935, 1958; Napalkov and Karas, 1957; Simonson and Brožek, 1959). Once the animal is conditioned, generalization of the conditioned stimulus (Cs) readily occurs; blood pressure elevations occur when the experimenter enters the laboratory, when the animal anticipates the conditioning procedure, or when the animal is strapped in the laboratory chair in which it sat before or during the training procedure. Based on such observations, Miasnikov (1954) has formulated the hypothesis that essential hypertension is a "conditioned neurosis" that has become generalized to many environmental stimuli. Once developed, the conditioned elevations are retained for many months (Dykman and Gantt, 1960).

Conditioning experiments are successful in monkeys and dogs but are less successful in cats (Shapiro and Horn, 1955). Mararychev and Kuritsa (1951) used injections of epinephrine as the Us, and a tone as the Cs to produce elevations in dogs. Renin has also been used as the Us (Andreev et al., 1952).

In some animals species, but not in others, both simple and complex unconditioned stimuli produce elevated levels of blood pressure. "Audiogenic" hypertension has been produced in rats by daily exposure to air blasts (Aceto et al., 1963; Farris et al., 1945; Rothlin et al., 1953). "Audiogenic" seizures produced by air blast may be accompanied by elevations of blood pressure in some rat strains and not in others: the predisposition to seizures is an inherited trait (Morgan and Galambos, 1942).

Pickering (1961) quoted a Russian experiment carried out by Miminoshvili (1960) in which a male monkey developed elevated arterial pressure and died after he was separated from his mate, who was put into an adjacent cage with another male monkey. Lapin (1965) and Miasnikov (1962) have confirmed this observation.

Not all animals develop high blood pressure when separated or exposed to simple stimuli, such as electric shock or loud noises. A combination of stimuli may have to be used. Shapiro and his co-workers (1955, 1957a) found that in rats, a combination of the experimental production of "anxiety" and the restriction of renal blood flow on one side after the removal of the other kidney caused hypertension to appear sooner and produced more-severe renal lesions than when rats were not made "anxious."

When rats are exposed to a light that warned of an impending electric shock to produce "conditioned emotional responses (CER)," transient pressor responses occur. Elevated blood pressure levels produced by injecting animals with angiotensin II could be further increased by producing a CER (Sapira et al., 1966).

Other types of conditioning procedures besides the CER elicit circulatory responses and also affect the animal's behavior in general (Figar, 1965; Gavlichek, 1952). Experimentally conditioned emotional responses, such as fear, alter the behavior of an animal even when it is not exposed to the conditioning procedure (Asafov, 1958; Gantt, 1958; Reese and Dykman, 1960). These unconditioned responses gradually disappear. Conditioned cardiovascular responses, such as elevations of blood pressure, can still be elicited experimentally for many years, even after the emotional, motor, or salivary responses that originally accompanied the circulatory responses can no longer be elicited (Froňková et al., 1957; Gantt, 1958).

Direct brain stimulation has also been used either as the Cs or the Us. Motor cortical area stimulation (as a Us) that does not produce muscular movements leads to vasoconstriction or vasodilation; parietal lobe stimulation leads only to vasoconstriction. When the Us is applied to one cortical site and the Cs to another, only vasoconstriction is produced in dogs (Orlov, 1959). These dogs develop hypertension that progressively becomes more severe over a period of months; the blood pressure remains elevated despite the fact that the conditioning procedures had previously been stopped (Froňková et al., 1959; Gantt, 1960). The hypertension is associated with pathological changes in the kidney. But not every animal subjected to conditioned brain stimulation develops high blood pressure or renal lesions—individual differences in blood pressure elevations are observed (Gantt, 1960).

Operant or conditioned avoidance procedures, not only classical conditioning, cause the blood pressure of monkeys to increase. Avoidance training carried out for a period of 15 days causes an initial acute rise and then a fall in both blood pressure and pulse rate. After the initial period of training, a continuous avoidance schedule is eventually associated with sustained increases in blood pressure. The level of blood pressure attained depends on the duration and complexity of the training schedule. When monkeys are placed on complex schedules, high blood pressure levels are sustained even when the monkey does not press a lever to avoid a shock (Forsyth, 1968). Systolic and diastolic blood pressures are raised continually after 7 to 12 months of daily avoidance conditioning lasting 12 hours a day. After months of avoidance conditioning, the animals also became more excitable and active. Pressor responses occur in response to many different stimuli, such as noises that had been "neutral" before training. In these experiments, there appeared to be no consistent relationship between the number of electric shocks the animal received, the animal's bar-pressing to avoid them, and the level of blood pressure attained.

It seems hard to understand why the acute elevations of blood pressure that had occurred in the first 15 days of this experiment then subsided, and that it took another 7 to 12 months for permanent hypertension to become established. It is possible that two separate mechanisms are responsible for the initial and the later increase in blood pressure levels. But we do not know what the nature of these two mechanisms is.

Forsyth's results in Rhesus monkeys have been verified in other laboratories and with other species of monkeys (Anderson and Brady, 1971, 1973; Benson et al., 1969, 1970; Herd et al., 1969). Benson and co-workers (1969) trained squirrel monkeys on a fixed-ratio schedule to turn off a light signaling painful shock. In four of six monkeys, elevations of mean arterial blood pressure ensued before, during, and after the experimental periods. Sustained blood pressure elevations were also obtained by changing the method, so that increases in the blood pressure would turn off the light and avert delivery of the shock. When a fall in blood pressure was used to control the signal and the electric shock, sustained decreases in blood pressure were obtained. Anderson and Brady (1973) reported on the cardiovascular effects of free-operant shock-avoidance in dogs. During the period before the experimental session, the blood pressure rose and the heart rate fell. During the session, both increased.

Until recently, studies on the conditioning of autonomic—and more specifically of cardiovascular—responses, were fraught with uncertainties. It has been argued that autonomic components of a conditioned response might result from an increase in muscular activity (Smith, 1954). Since no attempt had been made to put this issue to a test, this criticism lingered on until Miller and his co-workers (1969) disposed of it by paralyzing rats with curare and then conditioning them. They produced exquisite differential autonomic vasomotor responses, including increases and decreases in systolic blood pressure. These investigators also showed that glomerular filtration rate, renal blood flow, and urine formation can be altered by conditioning. These experiments have opened up a new area of investigation which has direct relevance for our understanding of hypertension (Folkow, 1971).

The use of conditioning procedures is not the only method of producing elevation of blood pressure. Immobilizing animals repeatedly for two weeks does so also. (This technique also produces gastric ulceration in the rat.) After a fortnight of daily restraint-immobilization, blood pressure levels are significantly elevated (50 mm Hg). Because serum levels of the enzyme DBH also rise after immobilization, the blood pressure increase is probably due to enhanced peripheral sympathetic activity. Two additional weeks of daily immobilization for two hours increases blood pressure and enzyme levels further. When the procedure is stopped, the blood pressure takes three weeks to fall to baseline levels, but serum levels of the enzyme become normal after five days, suggesting that blood pressure levels are sustained by some mechanism besides increased sympathetic activity (Lamprecht et al., 1973).

The evidence derived from studies on the conditioning of high blood pressure in animals is quite convincing. Blood pressure increases, changes in vasomotor tone, and other physiological variables that have been implicated in the pathogenesis of essential hypertension in man can be brought about by a variety of experimental techniques in the controlled setting of the laboratory. The recent studies by Mason (1968) and by Miller (1969) raise the exciting possibility that we may be on the verge of a major increase in knowledge about the factors and mechanisms that initiate essential hypertension and sustain high blood pressure. The experimental, in contrast to the clinical, evidence is much more convincing that environmental and "psychological" factors do influence blood pressure regulation by their impact on the brain. However, some may argue that these experimental studies, despite their elegance, are laboratory artifacts. They are not natural experiments because avoiding painful shock or being restrained is not the customary experience of animals. These studies need therefore to be supplemented by more naturalistic ones.

Hypertension Produced by Social Manipulation

THE ROLE OF PRIOR EXPERIENCE AND OF FIGHTING

The most convincing and systematic study of the role of natural and social experiences that produce prolonged systolic hypertension has been carried out in mice by Henry et al. (1967). Mixing male mice from different boxes, aggregating them in small boxes, exposing mice to a cat for 6 to 12 months, and producing territorial conflict in colonies of mixed males and females results in sustained elevations of systolic blood pressure, which are higher in male than in female mice. Henry and his co-workers (1967) also found that castrated male mice show minimal elevations in blood pressure when crowded into small boxes. Reserpine, but not anesthesia, also lowers sustained blood pressure elevations. When young mice are raised together, rather than apart, and are later crowded together or made to fight for territory, food, and females, their blood pressure does not show the increases seen in those brought up in isolation from weaning to maturity. Previously isolated mice with high levels of blood pressure were also found to have an interstitial nephritis after they died.

Henry (1971a, b) and his co-workers later worked out the mechanisms of the hypertension and interstitial nephritis in their mice. Socially isolated mice first show a decreased activity of tyrosine hydroxylase (TH) and phenylethanolamine N-methylatransferase (PNMT) activity in the adrenal gland. But the activity of both enzymes and of monoamine oxidase, and the levels of norepinephrine and epinephrine become elevated in animals that are subsequently stimulated by contact with other animals. The mechanisms of these increases was worked out by Thoenen and co-workers (1969). A reflex increase of sympathetic nerve activity on stimulation transsynaptically induces enzyme activity in the adrenal gland after a period of one to three days. Adrenal TH activity decreases after the splanchnic (sympathetic) nerve to the adrenal gland is cut. Therefore, the increase in TH activity in the adrenal gland is due to increased sympathetic activity and not increased pituitary or adrenocortical steroid activity.

Other experiments show that social stimulation (such as fighting) may increase the levels of adrenocortical steroids (Bronson, 1967; Christian et al., 1965), constrict renal vessels (Bing and Vinthen-Paulsen, 1952), and raise levels of epinephrine, norepinephrine, and serotonin in the brain (Welch and Welch, 1965, 1971). In mice, daily fighting that is sustained for 14 days induces elevations of brain catecholamine levels, and levels of epinephrine (but not norepinephrine) in the adrenal glands, causes the kidneys to be "shrunken and contracted," and the adrenals, hearts, and spleens to be enlarged.

Although there is much controversy among behavioral scientists about what constitutes aggression, an aggressive act in animals, and hostility in man, a considerable body of information has recently been accumulated by behavioral biologists about the physiology of fighting among animals, about fighting among animals for their territorial rights, the effects of crowding, the establishment of dominance and submission patterns, and the results of rearing animals alone and then later bringing them together. Ethological techniques are used to study the effects on the behavior of animals subjected to these procedures. By using these techniques, Henry's and his co-workers' studies have thrown light on the development of high blood pressure and renal disease in mice. They and others have also elucidated some of the biochemical mechanisms in the adrenal gland and brain that may bring about elevated blood pressure levels and renal disease.

In these studies the effect of prior experience on the neurochemistry of the brain has been studied. Socially isolating young animals alters the mean levels of various catecholamines, indoleamines, and amino acids as well as their biosynthetic and degradative enzymes in the brain (Welch and Welch, 1968b, 1971). Rearing young rodents in social isolation also alters the animals' reaction to various changes in their environment, their dominance and submission patterns in their social group, and their aggressive behavior. During the change from previous isolation to group living, marked changes occur in levels and turnover rates of both substrate and the enzyme levels in the brain.

Not all members of an animal genus or species are temperamentally aggressive: strain differences occur. Bourgault and co-workers (1963), and Karczmar and Scudder (1967) contrasted one aggressive strain of mice with a more peaceful strain. The brains of the aggressive mice contained lower levels of brain serotonin and norepinephrine. Subsequently, it was found that the content of biogenic amines in the brains of mice of different aggressive strains was not the same. In some aggressive strains, Maas (1962) found low levels of serotonin in the brain stem. In other strains, brain stem levels of serotonin are normal, but forebrain levels are low (Lagerspetz et al., 1967). When serotonin synthesis is inhibited by parachlorphenylalanine, nonaggressive mice kill members of their own species (Karli, 1969). Other mice of the same strain become killers when norepinephrine biosynthesis is inhibited by α-methylparatyrosine (Leaf, 1969). Therefore, the depletion of serotonin and of norepinephrine may cause some strains of mice to become killers. However, this effect cannot be the final answer to the problem of muricide because reserpine, which also depletes the brain of serotonin and norepinephrine, sedates animals. Sedated mice do not kill members of their species. The effects of inhibiting the synthesis of serotonin and norepinephrine by parachlorphenalanine and α-methylparatyrosine also produces exploratory behavior in addition to muricide. So far, we have no explanation for observations of this kind because a change in the level of a single neurotransmitter produces changes in a number of complex behaviors such as muricide or exploration.

It is easier to understand that early experience may lower the levels of an enzyme in the brain. Low levels of neuronal discharge in turn produce low levels of neurotransmitter biosynthesis and their biosynthetic products. Henry's (1967, 1969, 1971a, b) and the Welches' work (1971) can be understood in this context. When placed in a new and unfamiliar environment that provides excessive and unfamiliar stimulation, both aggressive behavior and increases in blood pressure occur because sensory stimulation is suddenly increased. As a consequence, a precipitous increase in the biosynthesis of neurotransmitter substances occurs.

Some support for this statement lies in the observation that male mice that had previously been isolated fought when they were individually paired with another mouse in an unfamiliar environment. The speed with which the fighting occurred and the duration and intensity of the fight was directly related to the length of prior isolation (Welch and Welch, 1971). Mice brought up together in groups took a much longer time to start a fight; the latent period before the onset of fighting depended on the number of peers in the group in which they had been raised (Welch and Welch, 1966, 1971). Both Henry and his co-workers (1967, 1969, 1971a, b) and Welch and Welch (1971) have found that prior isolation not only led to increased fighting when such animals are exposed to other animals, but also led them to assume a dominant role in the social hierarchy to which they have been introduced. Previously isolated animals even defeat a dominant animal that had been raised in a group (Welch and Welch, 1971).

Fighting produces peripheral sympathetic activation when the fight is intense. A reduction of epinephrine stores in the adrenal galnd and of levels of norepinephrine and dopamine in the brain stems of fighting rats and mice occurs (Vogt, 1954; Welch and Welch, 1971). A direct manner of measuring the level of peripheral sympathetic activation is to determine levels of DBH, the enzyme that converts dopamine into norepinephrine. The enzyme levels can be determined in different strains of rats, including those predisposed to hypertension, before and after a fight. In nonhypertensive strains of rats, the end of a fight is associated with a fall in blood pressure. But in spontaneously hypertensive rats and in salt-sensitive hypertensive and salt-resistant rats a fall in blood pressure levels does not occur after a fight. Animals in which a fall in blood pressure occurs after a fight have high initial levels of the enzyme: the higher the level of enzyme before the fight, the greater the fall in blood pressure after the fight. Therefore, a *decreased* peripheral sympathetic activity is associated with a failure of blood pressure to fall after fighting and characterizes strains of rats prone to hypertension (Lamprecht et al., 1974). These studies suggest that hypertensive strains of rats have a decreased peripheral sympathetic activity during and after a fight. Fighting does not change the blood pressure levels of hypertensive rats, because peripheral sympathetic activity remains unchanged during the fight. These results can be understood in only one way. During the inception of high blood pressure levels, peripheral sympathetic activity may be increased, but as soon as high blood pressure levels are established the activity may decrease and be unresponsive to fighting. In normal animals, by comparison, fighting causes a considerable fluctuation of sympathetic activity.

The observations suggest that marked individual differences in behavior and blood pressure levels occur in different strains of rodents when made to fight. In addition, the prior experience of a rodent determines its behavioral response. Rodents that are isolated when young fight more and assume the dominant role when they rejoin their group. They pay the price for their aggressive and assertive behavior by developing high blood pressure and interstitial nephritis. Their aggressive behavior is in some way functionally related to marked changes in the levels of enzymes involved in the biosynthesis of catecholamines in the brain. Levels of the enzymes in the brain are initially lower in animals isolated from the time of weaning but increase dramatically and excessively when the animals rejoin their group. Even when the animals have not previously been isolated, fighting changes levels of brain catecholamines. Furthermore, animals who are mere spectators to a fight and not participants in it, show changes in norepinephrine levels in the brain stem (Welch and Welch, 1968b, c, 1969).

Much has been learned about the complex interaction of strain differences, early experience, aggressive behavior, and high blood pressure from these studies. These experiments establish a relationship between aggressive or assertive behavior and high blood pressure in certain strains of animals. The relationship of aggression and high blood pressure has also been described in human beings. In animals this relationship seems to be mediated by changes in biogenic amine levels in the brain. Biogenic amines in the brain are organized in finite systems that also have an integral place in the regulation of arterial blood pressure (Chalmers, 1975). Indeed, strains of animals prone to hypertension differ from normotensive strains in the manner in which central monoaminergic systems are organized. These differences manifest themselves in the manner in which monoaminergic metabolism is organized in hypertensive and normotensive animals.

Genetic Factors and Experimental Hypertension in Animals

Early and later social experiences in mice not only cause high blood pressure but also influence behavior. The results of these experiments support the idea that social experiences can play a role in the initiation of high blood pressure. But the role of genetic factors in the establishment of hypertension in these mice was not determined. Other experiments clearly indicate that rodents vary in their predisposition to high blood pressure. Some strains develop high blood pressure spontaneously, other strains only do so when fed salt. Even in the former, the exact level of the blood pressure can be set by varying the amount of salt in the diet; in these animals, dietary salt does not initiate high blood pressure but determines its level. No experiment has been done to date in order to determine whether social experiences accelerate or retard the "spontaneous" develop-

47

ment of high blood pressure in either strain, although we do know that different strains of rats develop high blood pressure in different ways. For example, Smirk and Hall (1958) bred Wistar rats selectively for high blood pressure. The male rats in the group had higher resting blood pressure levels than the female rats. Both sexes responded with brisker blood pressure responses to the administration of drugs that produce pressor responses than did the normotensive rats. Their hearts weighed more and were frequently hypertrophic. Their heart rates under light anesthesia were higher, and some were found to have arteriolar necrosis. In young "hypertensive" rats, no arteriolar lesions occurred in the kidney. The peripheral resistance was increased in the hind-leg blood vessels of these hypertensive animals by neurogenic mechanisms. Both adrenalectomy and hyophysectomy reduced blood pressure levels. Therefore, adrenal or pituitary hormones may have contributed to the hypertension. Many of the hormones could have done so, but vasopressin was not one of them (Laverty and Smirk, 1961). Another strain of rats was bred by Okamoto and Áoki (1963) and Okamoto (1969). These rats developed hypertension "spontaneously" by a polygenic mechanism at about the age of 10 to 12 weeks. Although hypertension does develop when the rats are fed a salt-free diet (170 mm Hg), the amount of salt intake determines the level of the mean arterial pressure attained (to 230 mm Hg on 4% NaCl). Increasing the amount of potassium in the diet, which promotes sodium excretion, reduces the blood pressure levels (Louis et al., 1971). The spontaneously hypertensive strain of rats differs from the strain described by Dahl (see below) in that the former develop hypertension despite the absence of salt, as well as renal, cardiac, and cerebrovascular lesions that are akin to those in human hypertensive disease.

Spontaneously hypertensive rats show physiological variations from the norm even before hypertension begins. In spontaneously hypertensive rats of 8 weeks of age, plasma renin levels are similar to those in normotensive controls. Between 12 and 35 weeks of age, these rats have elevated plasma renin activity (DeJong et al., 1972; Sen et al., 1972). And Sinaiko and Mirkin (1974) have shown that kidney renin activity progressively increases in spontaneously hypertensive and control normotensive rats from the eighteenth day of fetal life until the first day of neonatal life. But in one-day old spontaneously hypertensive animals renin activity is significantly higher than in the control animals of the same age; the activity continues to be higher until the rats are 21 days old. By then the kidney renin activity in the normotensive animals has also increased, but now a fall in renin activity occurs only in the spontaneously hypertensive rat, only to increase again later.

A variety of other disturbances occur in these rats. Folkow and his co-workers (1973) subjected a pair of rats, one belonging to the spontaneously hypertensive strain and the other to a normotensive strain, to flashes of light, intermittent sound and vibration and measured their blood pressures and heart rates. Young (prehypertensive) and old (hypertensive) rats of the spontaneously hypertensive strain responded with greater and longer-lasting increases of blood pressure and heart rates, due to an increase in β-adrenergic activity, with sensory stimulation than did normotensive rats. Therefore, prehypertensive rats of the spontaneously hypertensive strain are predisposed to react to sensory stimuli by an increased β-adrenergic sympathetic activity that these investigators ascribe to a greater readiness for the mobilization of the defense alarm reaction. Pfeffer and Frohlich (1973) have also demonstrated that the heart rate, cardiac output, and arterior flow rates are increased during the inception of hypertension (at 10–12 weeks of age) in spontaneously hypertensive rats. The cardiac activity is significantly greater in 10- to 12-week old hypertensive rats than in normotensive rats of the same age. But both groups of rats of this age have a normal peripheral resistance. Later, in those rats in whom hypertension is established, the cardiac output is normal and the peripheral resistance is heightened. (The analogy of this form of spontaneous rat hypertension to some instances of human labile and later stable hypertension is striking because both initially have elevated heart rates and cardiac outputs but a normal peripheral resistance.)

Other physiological studies carried out on spontaneously hypertensive rats describe the sequence of events that accompany the development of high blood pressure. Folkow and co-workers (1970) found that despite complete relaxation of the arterioles, the resistance to blood flow in the systemic vascular bed relative to the perfusion pressure was higher in spontaneously hypertensive than in normotensive rats. But the resistance to flow in the renal vessels was *lower* in the spontaneously hypertensive rats, though the renal vessels themselves were less distensible. Because the resistance to flow in the kidney is lower than is usual, the high blood pressure in these animals is probably not initiated by the kidney. Rather, the increased resistance to flow in the rest of the circulation may produce the elevated blood pressure levels (Folkow, 1971). Folkow (1971) believes that the changes in resistance to flow in the systemic blood vessels in these animals is due to increased sympathetic nervous system activity. The increased activity may be produced by increased angiotensin II levels in the central nervous system. But Folkow's suggestion may not be correct because Williams and co-workers (1972b) found that the spontaneously hypertensive rats had significantly lower serum levels of DBH than normotensive, age-matched controls of the N.I.H.-Wistar strain, both before and after the development of the elevated blood pressures. As DBH levels reflect overall peripheral sympathetic activity, the lower levels in hypertensive rats suggest decreased, not increased, sympathetic activity.

Folkow has also suggested that the central nervous system participates in the pathogenesis of the high blood pressure in spontaneously hypertensive rats. Norepinephrine and aromatic L-amino acid decarboxylase levels are significantly reduced in the lower brain stem and hypothalamus of spontaneously hypertensive rats, when compared with a control group of normal animals (Yamori et al., 1970). But these determinations were made after the experimental group of animals had become hypertensive; therefore, the reduced levels might be the consequence of the high blood pressure levels. In fact, more recent studies did not confirm this finding (Nakamura et al., 1971).

The failure to reproduce these findings highlights the scientific problem that has repeatedly been mentioned throughout this chapter: the pathophysiological changes produced by high blood pressure levels must be separated from the antecedent physiological causes of hypertension. The best illustration of this thesis is that injections of 6-hydroxydopamine into the lateral ventricles of young rats of the spontaneously hypertensive strain prevents the development of elevated blood pressure levels (Finch et al., 1972). The intraventricular injection of 6-hydroxydopamine, which causes degeneration of catecholaminergic (noradrenergic and dopaminergic) nerve endings in the brain and depletion of their transmitter stores, does not lower high blood pressure levels once they are established in this strain of rats (Haeusler et al., 1972). Therefore, noradrenergic and dopaminergic neurons in the brain may play a role in the initiation of, but do not seem to play a role in the maintenance of, high blood pressure. Once established, the high levels may be maintained by serotonergic neurons in the brain. Parachlorphenylalanine, which reduces serotonin synthesis, also reduces high systolic blood pressure in this strain of rats (Jarrot et al., 1975).

Brain stem levels of the catecholamines may also be affected by stress that changes levels or turnover rates of brain monoamines. Although the manner in which stress alters levels and turnover rates of these putative neurotransmitters is unknown, recent experiments suggest that changed levels of brain monoamines are due to the complex interaction of stress, genetic endowment, and the previous experience of an animal. Welch and Welch (1968a) found that restraint stress—which can cause some rats to become hypertensive—of various durations raises the brain levels of norepinephrine, dopamine, and serotonin. The release of these substances from neurons is accelerated by sensory stimulation (Glowinski and Baldessarini, 1966; Norberg, 1967). Their decline in levels after pharmacological inhibition of their biosynthesis depends on the nature of the stimulus (Andén et al., 1966; Gordon, et al., 1966; Hillarp et al., 1966). In some circumstances and rat strains, monoamine concentrations in the brain are actually lowered by stress (Andén et al., 1966; Bliss and Zwanziger, 1966; Gordon et al., 1966; Maynert and Levi, 1964; Paulsen and Hess, 1963; Toh, 1960; Welch and Welch, 1968b). In other strains of rats, salt has been found to play a role in the pathogenesis of hypertension. Salt-sensitive strains of rats regularly develop hypertension on eating small amounts of salt, but it takes time (Meneely et al., 1954). Dahl et al. (1962, 1968), and Jaffe et al. (1969) reported that two genetic strains of rats exist; one strain is resistant to salt ingestion, and the other is sensitive to salt ingestion. Even a diet containing only 0.38 percent of salt causes salt-sensitive rats to have higher blood pressure levels (134 mm Hg, mean) than the salt-resistant ones (112 mm Hg, mean). Salt-resistant rats on a diet of 8 percent sodium chloride have no blood pressure increases, but the blood pressure of the salt-sensitive ones rises to 210 mm Hg on this excess of dietary salt, and they develop moderate to severe lesions of the kidneys. Moreover, even the sensitive rats on a low-salt diet showed changes in the musculoelastic arteriolar pads of the kidney. This anatomical lesion is thought to be inherited and not to be due to salt ingestion. The hypertensive tendency of the salt-sensitive strain can be transmitted to members of the salt-resistant strain by parabiosis (Dahl et al., 1969); presumably a humoral factor is responsible for transmission of the tendency to salt-sensitivity. Recent evidence suggests that transplanting a kidney from a salt-sensitive animal into a salt-resistant animal raises the latter's blood pressure—a result that suggests that the kidney produces a hypertensive substance (Dahl et al., 1972).

Salt-sensitive animals have low aldosterone output on a diet of salt (Rapp and Dahl, 1972). The reduction in aldosterone output may be one of several inherited tendencies that determine salt sensitivity for which a multigenic mode of inheritance has been demonstrated. One genetic locus with two alleles inherited by codominance accounts for 16 percent of the blood pressure differences between salt-sensitive and salt-resistant strains; it also accounts for an increased secretion of 18-OH desoxycorticosterone (Rapp and Dahl, 1971, 1972; Rapp et al., 1973). Other factors must account for the rest of the etiological variance. Williams and co-workers (1972b) reported lower serum levels of

DBH in the salt-sensitive strain than in salt-resistant animals. Animals made hypertensive by feeding salt and injecting desoxycorticosterone acetate also have low levels of DBH. And Iwai and co-workers (1973) found that the salt-sensitive strain of rats had low serum-renin activity and that the kidney contained low levels of renin. The amount of salt in the diet modifies the amount of serum renin activity, but serum renin activity level in blood remains lower on a high-salt diet in salt-sensitive rats when compared to members of the salt-resistant strain. Serum renin levels do not increase as much as expected when the renal artery is compressed on one side in salt-sensitive rats. Therefore, low renin levels in salt-sensitive rats may be an inherited characteristic.

Apparently, high blood pressure in salt-sensitive rats is not the product of any one factor. In fact, the level of blood pressure attained in these rats is not only determined by the amount of salt in the diet. Friedman and Dahl (1975) have shown that the blood pressure level attained can also be determined by a conflict situation that combines food deprivation and the application of electric shocks. Salt-sensitive rats exposed to this conflict develop a higher level of systolic blood pressure than rats of the same strain merely food deprived, or shocked without food deprivation. In some rats, the high levels of blood pressure after exposure to conflict persisted for three to four months. These experiments suggest that this strain of rats is as sensitive to psychological stress as it is to the amounts of salt in the diet and that high levels of blood pressure can be produced by both stress and salt.

Summary

High blood pressure may be initiated in the rat by a wide variety of techniques and experimental procedures and is not the product of any one "cause." There are many pathways by which the rat can develop high blood pressure. Different strains of rats may develop hypertension by different means: the salt-sensitive rat develops hypertension even when it ingests little salt, but the spontaneously hypertensive rat develops high blood pressure without salt, although the amounts of salt ingested determine the level of the high blood pressure. Environmental factors, stress, or salt ingestion determine the blood pressure level, and genetic factors determine the predisposition to hypertension. The genetic predisposition to hypertension is different in different strains of rats. The predisposition is multigenic and is expressed in different physiological disturbances. The work on genetic strains of rats that become hypertensive suggests that genetic heterogeneity exists. Hypertension can be produced by environmental manipulation in rats and mice without regard to inheritance. Henry's and the Welches' work highlights the importance of prior experience, of changing the ecological conditions, and of the roles of fighting and dominance patterns in the development of high blood pressure and renal disease in rodents. In addition, many different behavioral manipulations raise an animal's blood pressure. These manipulations consist of restraint-immobilization, excessive stimulation by noise, and conditioning techniques.

To summarize the results of investigations with animals: many different methods of inducing hypertension in animals have been successful. Experiments with the Goldblatt technique of producing hypertension suggest that the kidney has a self-regulating function in controlling the blood pressure—compression of one renal artery produces hypertension; when the other kidney is later removed, the blood pressure rises further, suggesting that prior to removal the second kidney suppressed the blood pressure.

Salt-feeding can produce sustained hypertension in some strains of rats. In part, this effect is mediated by increased mineralocorticoid (18-hydroxydesoxycorticosterone) production. In other rats, desoxycorticosterone acetate and aldosterone given with salt also produce experimental hypertension. Once hypertension is produced in this way and combined treatment is stopped, the blood pressure falls, only to increase again when only salt is fed. Presumably, different mechanisms are involved in initiating hypertension and producing its recurrence.

The spontaneously hypertensive rat is the best analog of human hypertension. Although differences between this animal model and the human disease exist (Okamoto, 1969), the similarities are striking. The elevation of blood pressure in the spontaneously hypertensive rat are age-related, for reasons that are still not understood, just as in human beings. Spontaneously hypertensive subjects could be studied serially in order to determine the physiological changes that precede the development of hypertension. The sequential changes could be compared with those that occur in other forms of hypertension in animals. Comparative studies of this kind could teach us that in different animal species, hypertension can develop by different mechanisms. In borderline or labile hypertension in man, or early in experimental hypertension in the dog, the cardiac output is raised, but the peripheral resistance is not (Coleman and Guyton, 1969). In dogs, an initial increase in cardiac output occurs followed sequentially by vasoconstriction and an increased peripheral resistance. In other forms of human hypertension, the cardiac output is normal initially, but the peripheral resistance is increased. It is probably premature to generalize too much from these findings to other species. Although in the dog an initial increase in cardiac output occurs, in other species the cardiac output may be normal at the beginning of experimental hypertension.

The physiological changes that occur early in experimental hypertension seem to differ in different species or in different members of the same species. Certainly different species have different physiological responses to the same experimental procedure. The same experimental procedure responded to differently may initiate hypertension by one set of mechanisms and sustain it by another set.

Experiments in rats seemed to have clarified a number of controversies. Different strains of rats develop hypertension by different mechanisms. In some strains, the tendency to high blood pressure is polygenically determined. In one strain, even small amounts of salt interact with multiple genetically determined variations to elicit the hypertensive tendency. But the level of the blood pressure attained is determined by the amount of salt in the diet or by stressful manipulations. In still other strains of rats, hypertension develops inevitably at a particular age, but the blood pressure levels can be manipulated by varying the amount of dietary salt. The development of hypertension in the spontaneously hypertensive strain can be prevented by injections of 6-hydroxydopamine into the brain. But once hypertension is established, injecting 6-hydroxydopamine into the brain does not lower the blood pressure. Therefore, different physiological mechanisms seem to be involved in the establishment and in the maintenance of hypertension in these rats.

THE PATHOPHYSIOLOGY OF ESSENTIAL HYPERTENSION

The psychological heterogeneity of patients with essential hypertension may reflect the physiological heterogeneity of the disease. The probable heterogeneity of the pathogenetic mechanisms of the disease is present in its very early phases (Eich et al., 1966; Freis, 1960; Julius and Schork, 1971). Behavioral scientists have generally not kept abreast of this fact. For many years they have been guided by a single concept—that all patients with essential hypertension have an unusual cardiovascular reactivity and that essential hypertension is a product of an increased peripheral resistance. They have tried to correlate emotional and other psychological states with the excessive vascular reactivity or with the increase in peripheral resistance. They have asked how inhibited anger or rage raises blood levels by raising the peripheral resistance. But the cardiac output and not the peripheral resistance is elevated in the early phases of some forms of disease.

Behavioral scientists have proceeded on the assumption that anger or rage must raise blood pressure levels (choleric people do get red in the face!). They have not considered that in essential hypertension, the anger might be the product of the increased blood pressure levels or reflect some underlying physiological change that is also expressed in high blood pressure. Until we have a way of predicting people who will develop essential hypertension, these alternative possibilities will continue to plague the behavioral scientist.

Progress in understanding essential hypertension occurs daily. One major advance has been made in specifying the physiology of the early phases of the disease.

The Role of the Cardiovascular System and the Circulation in Essential Hypertension

Early in the course of essential hypertension, a high cardiac output occurs in some young patients with borderline essential hypertension (Eich et al., 1966; Folkow, 1971; Tobian, 1972). The increased cardiac output is accompanied by a slight increase in peripheral resistance. After a time, the peripheral resistance rises further, and the cardiac output returns to normal levels (Freis, 1960; Guyton and Coleman, 1969). In these patients, the increases in peripheral resistance are secondary—the consequence of the increase in cardiac output. The reasons for the elevation of the cardiac output are not known. An initial increase in cardiac output may be due to an increase in extracellular fluid volume (Coleman and Guyton, 1969). On the other hand it may be due to increased β-adrenergic sympathetic stimulation of the heart.

The increase in cardiac output does not occur in all patients (Widimsky et al., 1957). It may depend on the patient's age (Julius and Conway, 1968; Lund-Johansen, 1967). In young patients the increased cardiac output at rest is of the order of 14 percent. An increased heart rate and oxygen consumption may also occur with an increased cardiac output. Later, when the peripheral resistance is increased and there is visible evidence of retinal arteriolar spasm, the cardiac output, heart rate, and oxygen consumption become normal. Once the peripheral resistance is increased, exercise causes the arterial blood pressure to rise. Cardiac output and stroke volume do not rise in borderline hypertensive patients or hypertensive patients with an increased peripheral resistance as much as in a normal group of subjects during exercise. But in both groups of hypertensive patients, exercise is associated with greater increases in peripheral resistance than in normal subjects (Sannerstedt, 1969). Some borderline hypertensive patients with an increased cardiac output have and some do not have an increased heart rate at rest (Bello et al., 1967; Finkielman et al., 1965). Propranolol does not reduce the elevated heart rate (Julius et al., 1968), but it does lower the cardiac output in borderline hypertensive patients (Julius et al., 1968; Ulrych et al., 1968). Therefore, the increased cardiac output is probably due to β-adrenergic stimulation of the heart.

In some animals, the constriction of one renal artery may at first produce an increase in cardiac output and blood pressure that are later followed by an increase in peripheral resistance (Bianchi et al., 1970; Ferrario et al., 1970; Frohlich et al., 1969; Ledingham, 1971). After a period of several weeks and further increases in blood pressure and peripheral resistance, the cardiac output settles back to normal levels. When the clamp on the renal artery is removed, a further temporary increase in peripheral resistance occurs, in the face of a prompt decrease in cardiac output and blood pressure. These hemodynamic responses, following the relief of renal artery constriction, can only, in part, be explained by changes in blood volume (Floyer, 1955).

The secondary increases in peripheral resistance seem to be the regulatory consequence of an increased cardiac output. When the output exceeds the metabolic requirements of local tissue, local vasoconstriction occurs, raising the peripheral resistance to lower the blood flow in that region of the body (Patterson et al., 1957). If the increase in peripheral resistance occurs throughout the body, the blood pressure increases and the cardiac output is reduced to normal. Regional differences in resistance to blood flow do occur in essential hypertension and in the experimental forms of hypertension produced by clamping a renal artery (Brod, 1970; Folkow, 1971; Rushmer, 1958). The causes of an increased cardiac output, experimentally produced in animals, are understood somewhat better than the causes of an increased cardiac output in some young male borderline hypertensives. (It is possible that the increased β-adrenergic stimulation of the heart can be related to emotional states that are mediated by the brain.)

Early in essential hypertension, physiological heterogeneity exists. In some patients both cardiac output and heart rate are increased; in others, only the cardiac output is elevated; in a third group the cardiac output is normal but the peripheral resistance is increased. In other hypertensive patients with established high blood pressure levels, the cardiac output may be lower than normal, even when no congestive heart failure is present. In these patients the high blood pressure and the low cardiac output do not respond to the stimulus of exercise.

FACTORS AFFECTING THE INCREASED PERIPHERAL RESISTANCE
IN ESSENTIAL HYPERTENSION

At some stage in essential hypertension the increased peripheral resistance is increased. It is not clear whether the increase precedes or follows the disease process in every form of essential hypertension. The enhanced peripheral resistance is due to constriction of the small arteries and veins—the so-called resistance vessels. The increase is not due to changes in blood viscosity, blood flow, or velocity profiles. The changes in the diameter of resistance vessels account for virtually all the changes in regional blood flow. Their reduced diameter is caused by local metabolic products and by adjustments in the tonic and phasic activity of sympathetic vasoconstrictor (or vasodilator) neurons, rather than by the action of the catecholamines (Celander, 1954). Adjustments in the ratio of resistance between the pre- and post-capillary bed affects the balance between the intravascular and extravascular body-water compartments that in turn affect the kidney (Rankin and Pappenheimer, 1957; Mellander, 1960). Regional blood volume and flow can change relatively independently of each other, by virtue of the design of resistance vessels. Major changes in blood flow in a region of the body can occur with only trivial changes in blood volume. Moderate increases in the tone of the smooth muscle in the vessel wall can occasion very large increments in the resistance to flow. Intrinsic myogenic activity in part determines such shifts that need not be produced by changes in vasomotor tone.

Peterson (1961) has suggested that in essential hypertension, excessive contraction of the smooth muscle wall of the resistance vessels causes increasd moduli of elasticity and viscosity. The increased stiffness of the resistance vessels is due to an increase in their water and electrolyte content. As they swell, their radius is reduced. The increased peripheral resistance may be due to local or systemic factors that account for the increase in peripheral resistance in essential hypertension.

Discharge in sympathetic vasodilator neurons may contribute to the increased peripheral resistance. These neurons are distributed to the arteriolar section of resistance vessels (Folkow et al., 1961; Uvnäs, 1960). They could account for the contraction of the vessels. But local tissue needs determine their own blood supply and the patency of vessels. No method has been developed for determining whether the increased vasoconstrictor tone in essential hypertension is due to changes in the chemical composition or structure of the arteriolar wall (Tobian and Binion, 1952; Tobian and Chesley, 1966; Tobian et al., 1961, 1969a), to the increased responsiveness of arteriolar muscle cells and their myogenic activity, to local tissue needs or to increased sympathetic discharge. In the rat the increase of peripheral resistance is caused by a change in the chemical composition of the arteriolar wall—a consequence of persistent hypertension. In man, the wall of the renal artery in hypertensive patients also contains an excess of sodium and water (Tobian and Binion, 1952).

We do not know which of these several possible causes of increased resistance comes first. It cannot be assumed, therefore, that the increased peripheral resistance in essential hypertension is only produced by increased sympathetic discharge. This assumption is based on the idea that increased sympathetic discharge mediates emotional changes in hypertensive persons.

Once changes in the arteriolar wall occur, the peripheral resistance may be affected in different ways. The narrowed arteriolar lumen may impede flow. The increased salt and water content of the wall may reduce the elasticity of the arteriole (Feigl et al., 1963). The increased sodium content of the arteriolar cell may diminish the intracellular content of potassium and lower its membrane potential to produce partial depolarization and contraction of the arteriolar smooth muscle (Emanuel et al., 1959). The increased intracellular content of free calcium may directly cause smooth muscle proteins to contract. These proteins are sensitized to calcium by the presence of sodium, whose content is increased within the arteriolar cell wall.

The increased content of water, sodium, and calcium may cause the wall to swell and produce mechanically and functionally an increased resistance to the flow of blood. The hypertrophy of muscle in the arteriolar wall also augments the resistance. The resistance changes must be viewed in dynamic terms of dilation or contraction that occur in the arteriolar vascular bed. In essential hypertension, the arterioles resist flow even under conditions of maximal dilatation (Folkow, 1971) presumably because they are thickened (Short, 1966) or "waterlogged."

When these arterioles are made to contract by the interarterial injection of norepinephrine, the resistance increases in hypertensive but not in normotensive humans (Doyle and Fraser, 1961) and in hypertensive rats. This effect is not only due to the drug but is also the product of the preexisting state of the arteriolar wall. Norepinephrine augments the resistance to flow because it causes further contraction of an already narrowed arteriole. On further contraction the slope of increase of resistance is much steeper for a thickened, contracted arteriole (Redleaf and Tobian, 1958b; Mendlowitz et al., 1959, 1961; Sivertsson, 1970; Folkow, 1971).

Therefore the reactivity of the arterioles to norepinephrine may be no different in hypertensive patients than in normals, but the state of the arterioles differs. Neurogenic vasoconstriction has been indirectly implicated as the cause of the increased peripheral resistance in essential hypertension because of the effects of sympathectomy and of antihypertensive drugs. The same dose of a drug has a greater depressor effect in hypertensive than in normotensive subjects (Arnold and Rosenheim, 1949). A drug like chlorothiazide increases the caliber of blood vessels (Hollander and Wilkins, 1957; Freis et al., 1958) and, therefore, reduces the effects of norepinephrine (Beavers and Blackmore, 1958). But the effects of drugs cannot be used to support the neurogenic vasoconstrictor hypothesis of essential hypertension because drugs that block ganglionic transmission also decrease cardiac output and lower the blood pressure.

Increased neurogenic vasoconstriction in essential hypertension has been more directly inferred from studies of the circulation of the fingers after injection of norepinephrine (Folkow, 1971; Mendlowitz et al., 1958; Mendlowitz and Naftchi, 1958). But the evidence for an increased sensitivity of the arterioles in the fingers of hypertensive patients is not clearcut.

Norepinephrine acts directly on the vessel wall of hypertensive animals and increases its stiffness tenfold (Peterson et al., 1961; Holloway et al., 1973). But the action of norepinephrine may be secondary to the presence of other factors in the disease, and may not be the initial reason for vasoconstriction. Sympathetic denervation or blockade of an area enhances the sensitivity of its blood vessels to norepinephrine. Infusion of angiotensin potentiates the effects of norepinephrine on blood vessels. Cortisone increases the sensitivity of blood vessels to norepinephrine (Mendlowitz et al, 1958, 1961), possibly by interfering with its enzymatic degradation (Mendlowitz et al., 1959). Norepinephrine may play a role in enhancing the peripheral resistance during the course of the disease by interacting with other factors, but may not initiate the original increase in peripheral resistance. The increased blood pressure in essential hypertension was formerly thought to be secondary to an increase in peripheral resistance. Actually the reverse may be correct. Thickening of blood vessel walls can be produced by experimentally raising the blood pressure in animals (Silvertsson, 1970; Folkow, 1971). The arteriolar wall thins out when the blood pressure is reduced to normal levels. Damage to large vessels such as the renal artery may result from high blood pressure (Shapiro et al., 1969). Once a renal artery is damaged, a vicious cycle is set up: essential hypertension may produce renovascular hypertension that sustains or augments preexisting high blood pressure levels. However, Tobian (1972) believes that thickened or damaged renal arterioles do not maintain high blood pressure levels by themselves. Recent evidence suggests that both the increased peripheral resistance and vascular damage are respectively the consequences of an increase in cardiac output and of high blood pressure levels in some patients with essential hypertension. They may help to sustain but not to initiate the disease.

The Role of the Kidney in Essential Hypertension

Because the kidney plays major roles in raising and lowering the blood pressure, it has also figured prominently in theories about the pathogenesis of essential hypertension. Constriction of the renal artery by various lesions and acute and chronic kidney diseases all elevate blood pressure. Some of the reasons for a narrowed renal artery may, however, stem from preexisting hypertension.

Ever since Goldblatt (1947) demonstrated that narrowing of one renal artery experimentally produces hypertension in animals, an enormous amount of investigative effort has been expended on the role of the kidney in the pathogenesis of essential hypertension and in maintaining normal blood pressure levels. When one renal artery is partly occluded, removal of the other kidney further enhances blood pressure levels (Goldblatt, 1947). Therefore, the normal kidney lowers.the blood pressure possibly by regulating the extracellular fluid volume. In the rat, even when the salt intake is restricted, clamping the renal artery on one side and removing the other kidney still produces further elevations of blood pressure levels (Redleaf and Tobian, 1958). Therefore, the blood pressure increases despite a stable extracellular fluid volume and without further increases of already elevated renin levels (Brown et al., 1966).

In sheep, extracellular fluid volume actually falls following constriction of one renal artery, but the blood pressure rises so that the increase in fluid volume cannot account for the hypertension. When both renal arteries are constricted, sodium is not conserved, so extracellular fluid volume is not increased, and the hypertension is due to the release of renin and the mobilization of the angiotensin-aldosterone system. Therefore, different mechanisms can make the blood pressure increase when different experimental techniques are used. Furthermore, different species respond in different ways to the same experimental procedure. In dogs, unilateral constriction of the renal artery is associated almost immediately by renin release and an increase in blood pressure that can be prevented by an enzyme inhibitor that is injected at the time the artery is clamped. But once high blood levels are established for a week by clamping the artery, the enzyme inhibitor no longer reduces the blood pressure—a result suggesting that two different mechanisms are sequentially involved in initiating and in sustaining elevations of the blood pressure (Gutmann et al., 1973; Miller et al., 1972).

After both the rat's kidneys are removed, the intake of large amounts of sodium and water—that increase the extracellular fluid volume—raises the blood pressure even further (Tobian, 1950). The antihypertensive function of the kidney is, therefore, only in part due to the excretion of excess salt and water.

In man, the normal kidney also has an antihypertensive function (Merrill et al., 1956). In the rat, a normal kidney implanted after renal artery constriction lowers the blood pressure, providing that the perfusion pressure of the new kidney is at high levels (Tobian et al., 1964). When the perfusion pressure is in the normal range the blood pressure remains high. The high perfusion pressure causes the normal kidney to release antihypertensive substances, possibly the prostaglandins.

When a renal artery is constricted experimentally or by disease, a fall in pressure occurs distal to the constriction. As a result of this pressure drop renin is released by the kidney and serum renin activity increases. The hypertensive effects of the kidney may be mediated by the renin-angiotensin mechanism (Tobian, 1960), but this hypothesis has been questioned, because a fall in blood pressure can be produced in rats and sheep even when their blood angiotensin and plasma renin levels remain unchanged (Blair-West et al., 1968a, b; Byrom and Dodson, 1949; Floyer, 1955). The acute fall in blood pressure after unclipping a renal artery may be due to reflex sympathetic discharge that raises the heart rate and maintains cardiac output to compensate for the fall in blood pressure. Because renin and angiotensin levels remain the same despite a fall in blood pressure they may not be essential to the maintenance of renovascular hypertension (Funder et al., 1970).

When antibodies to renin or angiotensin are administered to dogs or rats with a constricted renal artery, the increase in blood pressure levels is averted or the blood pressure, if already elevated, falls (Christlieb et al., 1969; Carretero et al., 1971). Other species, such as the rabbit, may respond differently. When the contralateral kidney is removed from a rabbit whose other renal artery was constricted, the antibodies to renin and angiotensin have no antihypertensive effect (Bing and Poulsen, 1970; Brunner et al., 1971; Christlieb et al., 1969). Presumably, a new mechanism, other than renin release, sustains blood pressure levels in the rabbit. Therefore, the conclusion can be reached that different mechanisms sustain high blood pressure in different species. And different species of animals respond to the same experimental techniques in a different manner.

THE CONTROL OF THE RENIN AND ANGIOTENSIN MECHANISMS

One of the major advances our understanding of the pathophysiology of essential hypertension has been the elucidation of the physiological mechanism by which the kidney and the enzyme renin are related to the adrenocortical mineralocorticoid, aldosterone, and to the formation of the polypeptides, angiotensin I and II. Renin release is controlled by interrelated regulatory mechanisms that influence the level of arterial pressure and, therefore, the pressure within the renal artery. A fall in renal artery perfusion pressure causes the increased production and secretion of renin by the granular, juxtaglomerular cells that lie within the walls of the afferent arterioles of the kidney (Tobian, 1960, 1962).

The exact mechanism by which a fall in perfusion pressure produces renin release is unknown. Vander and Miller (1964) do not believe that renin release is stimulated by the mechanical effect of a fall in renal artery pressure. Renin release can be ascribed to a reduction in the delivery of sodium to the macula densa portion of the distal renal tubules when the pressure falls. Eide and co-workers (1973), on the other hand, believe that renin release depends on the state of dilatation of the renal arterioles. Renin release would then be stimulated by the active dilatation of the renal arterioles in response to a fall in blood pressure—an autoregulatory process—rather than by reduced distension of the arteriolar wall. Once released, renin may act locally within the kidney to raise the blood pressure. It also enters the circulation directly or indirectly by way of the lymphatic system (Skinner et al., 1963). Renin converts the plasma globulin angiotensinogen into a decapeptide, angiotensin I, which further loses two amino acids, through the agency of an enzyme in the kidney, lung, and blood, to form the potent pressor substance angiotensin II. Angiotensin II acts on brain-stem pressor mechanisms and directly on arterioles to raise the blood pressure. As angiotensin II levels increase, the adrenocortical mineralocorticoid aldosterone is released. Angiotensin II is an important but not the only regulator of aldosterone secretion.

Renin may not be the only enzyme in the body to produce angiotensin I from the globulin substrate. An enzyme called tonin, found in the submaxillary gland, also converts angiotensin I into angiotensin II, but, unlike renin, it may produce the latter directly from globulin and from a 14-amino-acid polypeptide derived from the substrate (Boucher et al., 1974).

Although a fall in renal artery perfusion pressure is the main stimulus to renin release, a fall in plasma volume also causes its release. Conversely, increases in plasma volume or renal artery pressure inhibit renin release from the kidney (Tobian et al., 1964).

Adrenergic stimulation of the kidney also releases renin (Gordon et al., 1967). The effect is mediated by β-adrenergic receptors (Ganong, 1972). In the isolated rat kidney, isoproterenol stimulates renin release without changing renal artery perfusion pressure. The effect of isoproterenol is blocked by dipropananol. Norepinephrine also releases renin while causing renal artery vasoconstriction. When the vasoconstriction is averted by the appropriate blocking agent, renin release still occurs (Vandongen et al., 1973).

The sympathetic nervous system not only releases renin; it also exerts a resting, tonic effect on the juxaglomerular cells of the kidney. Renal sympathectomy decreases plasma renin activity (Mogil et al., 1969). Stimulation of the medulla oblongata increases it (Passo et al., 1971). Stimulation of the hypothalamus of the dog at various points —rostral to the preoptic area and ventral to the anterior commissure, at the level of the premammillary nucleus, and in the tuberal region—lowers plasma renin activity. Renal denervation prevents the fall in renin activity when the hypothalamus is stimulated. The pathways that mediate the effect of hypothalamic stimulation are not known. Hypothalamic stimulation at the same site also lowers the blood pressure, but not by altering renal blood flow (Zehr and Feigl, 1973). Therefore, the central nervous system may exert direct control on renin release and may be implicated in the pathogensis of essential hypertension.

The control of renin release after renal artery constriction may be more complicated and more individual than was once believed. After renal artery constriction some dogs develop elevated blood pressure levels, increased renin and aldosterone blood levels, and convulsions. In other dogs the levels of renin and aldosterone rise initially, then they fall, despite a permanent elevation of blood pressure (Brown et al., 1966; Carpenter et al., 1961b). The mechanisms whereby renin levels return to normal values in the second group of dogs have not been elucidated as yet.

In the second group of dogs, blood pressure levels are maintained in the face of normal serum renin activity. The lack of a correlation between blood pressure and renin levels occurs both in man and in dogs. Patients with essential hypertension may have low, normal, or high serum renin levels (Brunner et al., 1972). In dogs, arterial pressure levels do not correlate with serum renin levels; marked discrepancies and changes in renin levels occur (Ayers et al., 1969). In man, no linear relationship between blood pressure and renin levels occurs either, even in patients with essential or renovascular hypertension (Kaneko et al., 1967, 1968). The release of renin and the production of angiotensin II may occur at the inception of experimental hypertension in some animals, but high blood pressure levels are probably not sustained by increased renin or angiotensin II activity.

The role the renin-angiotensin-aldosterone system in the etiology and pathogenesis of essential hypertension remains enigmatic. In this disease, plasma renin levels may be low, normal, or high (Helmer, 1964; Creditor and Loschky, 1967; Ledingham et al., 1967; Jose et al., 1970; Brunner et al., 1972). High levels of renin and aldosterone activity in blood serum occur mainly in the malignant phase of the disease, when the kidney is damaged (Laragh, 1960, 1961; Laragh et al., 1972) or in Goldblatt hypertension and its natural analogues. The vascular lesions during the malignant phase of hypertensive disease may be directly due to the damaging effects of excessive renin and angiotensin activity on the walls of blood vessels (Carpenter et al., 1961b; Masson et al., 1962; Giese, 1964).

Of 219 patients with essential hypertension, 27 percent had reduced plasma renin activity when compared to normal volunteers. Of these patients, 16 percent had elevated levels of plasma renin, and 57 percent had normal levels. The amounts of aldosterone excreted by hypertensive patients vary more than in normal volunteers (Brunner et al., 1972). Black hypertensive patients are unusually likely to have a low serum renin activity despite the fact that they are more likely to develop malignant hypertension than white hypertensive patients. Patients with high serum renin activity have significantly higher mean diastolic blood pressures and blood urea nitrogen levels and lower plasma potassium levels, but suprisingly, their aldosterone levels are normal. Some (13–21 percent) of the patients with low serum renin activity had normal urinary aldosterone levels, which was unexpected. Only about 50 percent of all 219 patients with essential hypertension had preserved the usual linear relationshps between renin and aldosterone levels (Brunner et al., 1972).

These findings suggest that essential hypertension is a heterogeneous disease. In 50 percent of the patients, a disturbance in the regulation of aldosterone by angiotensin occurs. In other patients, the relationship between the two is retained. Heterogeneity is also suggested by the fact that essential hypertension can occur with every kind of serum renin activity—low, normal, and high. It remains to be shown whether variations in renin levels antecede the development of essential hypertension, are a correlate, or a result from it. Brunner et al. (1972) have found that renin levels remain the same in hypertensive patients over a period of months or years, suggesting that they are an abiding characteristic of these patients and do not result from some other variable, such as the disease process or elevated blood pressure levels. Renin levels may rise only when the malignant phase of the disease is ushered in.

THE PHYSIOLOGICAL ACTIONS OF ANGIOTENSIN

In normal subjects, angiotensin II infusion diminishes diuresis and produces sodium retention and an increased secretion rate of aldosterone and cortisol. Angiotensin II also stimulates ACTH secretion to increase cortisol production (Ames et al., 1965). The retention of sodium is brought about by direct stimulation of aldosterone secretion. Changes in cortisol production are also produced by mechanisms besides ACTH secretion. Fluctuations in levels of the glucocorticoids (such as cortisol) covary with changes in intravascular pressure, or an effective plasma volume (Ehrlich et al., 1966, 1967; Ehrlich, 1968; Kuchel et al., 1967). Patients with essential hypertension show no alterations in total exchangeable sodium, extracellular fluid, or plasma volume unless they are in congestive heart failure (Chobanian et al., 1961; Hollander and Wilkins, 1957). They paradoxically eliminate a greater proportion of a salt and water load after saline, water, or angiotensin infusion than normotensive subjects do (Baldwin et al., 1958; Cottier, 1960; Farnsworth, 1946; Green and Ellis, 1954; Hollander and Wilkins, 1957). The increased natriuresis and diuresis may be the result of the elevated blood pressure (Cottier, 1960) or of an increased tubular rejection of sodium that in turn depends on elevations of intrarenal pressure (Cottier, 1960). With a fall in blood pressure, regardless of what occasions it, the increased natriuresis and diuresis brought about by saline or water infusion diminishes.

The infusion of 5 mg of angiotensin II into patients with hypertension, regardless of pathogenesis, regularly produces an osmotic diuresis.* Increased amounts of electrolyte and water are excreted, even when no increases in blood pressure are produced by angiotensin. By contrast, 5 mg of angiotensin II produces an antidiuresis and a fall in electrolyte excretion in normal individuals (Bock and Krecke, 1958; Peart, 1959). When a renal artery stenosis is relieved and the blood pressure reverts to normal levels, the normal antidiuretic response to angiotensin infusion is reestablished (Peart, 1959).

The effect of angiotensin II on the excretion of salt and water depends on the level of the blood pressure. The paradoxical effect of angiotensin II on salt excretion may be an

---

* Osmotic diuresis also occurs with the "emotional effects" of passing a urethral catheter into women, when catheterization is followed by a discussion of their illness. Miles and De Wardener (1953) found that an increase in urine flow, chloride, and osmolar excretion rates occured in both hypertensive and normotensive patients. But the increases were considerably greater in the hypertensive than in the normotensive subjects. These authors also found that the increases mentioned often began before the catheter was actually inserted, but the specific emotional states of their subjects are not described in detail. They concluded that the mechanism of this osmotic diuresis was a diminished tubular reabsorption of salt. This experiment is important because it may account for the results obtained when mannitol, salt, or water are infused into hypertensive subjects.

adaptation to high blood pressure levels. If hypertensive patients eliminate more salt and water when angiotensin II or salt is infused, the blood pressure would be reduced.

The effects of angiotensin II can be understood in terms of physiological adaptation because the effect of any stimulus—in this instance angiotensin II—depends on the preexisting state, specifically whether blood pressure levels are elevated or not.

THE ROLE OF ANGIOTENSIN IN PRODUCING ELEVATED BLOOD PRESSURE

Angiotensin II has effects on the functions of the kidney, and it also has powerful pressor effects. Angiotensin II constricts arterioles directly, and also reflexly produces vasoconstriction by its effects on the pressor mechanisms in the brain stem. It stimulates aldosterone secretion thereby producing salt retention, which elevates the blood pressure (Carpenter et al., 1961b). Angiotensin II indirectly produces an increase in the sodium content of the arteriolar wall. It stimulates the release of norepinephrine from sympathetic postganglionic neurons and the adrenal medulla, and it potentiates the vasoconstrictor action of norepinephrine. Hypertensive patients may be sensitized by angiotensin II to overreact physiologically to psychological stimuli once the disease process has begun. Psychological stimuli may, therefore, aggravate the disease. In support of this hypothesis McCubbin (1967) has found that after very small doses of angiotensin II, which had no immediate effect on blood pressure levels, had been infused for several days into dogs, the arterial blood pressure became elevated and labile. When the dogs were surrounded by everyday activity in the laboratory, the arterial pressures were labile and high. If the laboratory was quiet, minor distractions caused marked further increases in arterial pressure. After the injection of angiotensin II the dogs became sensitized to the administration of tyramine, which releases endogenous stores of norepinephrine. Tyramine injection produced further elevations of the dogs' arterial pressures. The results of McCubbin's experiments strongly suggest that angiotensin II plays a role in the initiation of high blood pressure levels and alters the reactivity of the animal to environmental stimuli. Once these changes have occurred, the animal overreacts even to trivial stimuli. Environmental stimuli or drugs, such as tyramine, produce excessive responses that did not occur before treatment with angiotensin II. Therefore, one may conclude that psychological stimuli do not necessarily initiate high blood pressure levels. Angiotensin II alters the reactivity of dogs to environmental stimuli by mechanisms that may include the effects of angiotensin II on the brain. It may alter the function of the brain so that it responds in new ways to environmental stimuli by changing levels or turnover rates of brain catecholamines (Chalmers, 1975).

Angiotensin II amide in very small amounts acts directly on certain regions of the brain. It increases water drinking in rats who are in normal fluid balance without raising the blood pressure. Repetitive brain injections continue to produce the effect on drinking. Injections also wake up the sleeping rat. They interrupt eating in hungry rats and cause them to drink. Angiotensin II acts on the anterior hypothalamus and the preoptic and septal areas of the brain to produce drinking. Injections of angiotensin elsewhere in the brain do not produce drinking. The effect of angiotensin II on drinking behavior can also be produced by renin and carbachol (Booth, 1968; Epstein et al., 1970), but the effects of angiotensin II are more potent. Lehr and his co-workers (1973) believe that angiotensin I is as potent as angiotensin II in producing drinking in the rat. Drinking water is also usually accompanied by salt intake. If excessive amounts of water are drunk or salt is eaten, the extracellular fluid volume of the organism would increase and the blood pressure would rise.

The fact that injecting renin into the hypothalamus also produces drinking suggests that renin substrate is present in the brain. In fact, renin isoenzymes have been isolated from the brain, so that it is possible that the brain is itself capable of manufacturing angiotensin I or II. Angiotensin II levels are elevated in the cerebrospinal fluid (CSF) of the spontaneously hypertensive rat—the best animal model of essential hypertension in man. Antibodies against angiotensin II administered to these rats lowers their blood pressure (Ganten et al., 1974). But we do not know whether the angiotensin II in the CSF of these rats comes from brain or kidney renin activity.

THE PROSTAGLANDINS AS NATURALLY OCCURRING ANTIHYPERTENSIVE AGENTS

The kidney not only produces substances, such as renin, that are indirectly involved in raising blood pressure, but it also produces substances that lower it. In short, the kidney contains an autoregulatory mechanism for the control of blood pressure. The antihypertensive substances are produced by cells in the renal medulla (Muirhead et al., 1970). Removal of these cells causes the blood pressure to increase. The renal medullary cells of the rabbit contain prostaglandin E_2 (PGE2) (Hickler et al., 1964; Lee et al., 1966; Muirhead et al., 1967; Strong et al., 1966). Injections of PGE2 lower the blood pressure in normal and hypertensive rats. Other antihypertensive lipids have also been isolated from the renal medulla. They, too, lower the blood pressure of animals after constriction of one renal artery (Muirhead et al., 1967).

A third substance, polypeptide in nature, has been isolated from the aorta of dogs and from human and canine plasma. It also rapidly reduces blood pressure levels when injected into rats. Plasma levels of the polypeptide are increased in human beings and dogs with low blood pressure levels caused by surgical or experimental shock (Rosenthal et al., 1973). Still other hypotensive substances are released by shock and may account for the reduced blood pressure levels in shock (Lefer, 1973).

Antihypertensive substances such as PGE2 play a role in experimental hypertension in animals. It is as yet too early to say what the role of these substances is in human essential hypertension or in its treatment; little is known about the mechanisms regulating their synthesis, release, or secretion, or how they may interact with the various other regulators of blood pressure.

The Role of Salt and Water Metabolism in Essential Hypertension

INTRODUCTION

The maintenance of normal blood pressure levels in man depends in part on the volume of circulating blood. If hemorrhage occurs, the blood volume diminishes and the blood pressure falls. As the blood pressure falls a large number of mechanisms are brought into action to maintain the normal or raise the fallen blood pressure levels. Physiological readjustments occur to restore the blood volume. The fluid contained in the blood vessels constitutes only one part of all the fluid in the tissue spaces between cells. The extracellular fluid volume of the body is made up of all the fluid within blood vessels and outside cells in tissue spaces. The fluids in tissue spaces and in the blood vessels are in dynamic equilibrium with each other. As hemorrhage occurs, the fluid shifts out of tissue spaces into blood vessels to increase the blood volume. As the blood volume diminishes with hemorrhage, thirst promotes the drinking of water and intake of salt.

If the extracellular fluid volume is too large, or the osmotic pressure of the fluid is increased by salt, the body rids itself of water and salt respectively to maintain a relatively constant fluid volume and osmotic pressure. A number of interrelated mechanisms are involved in maintaining the equilibrium between fluid volume and salt content. The kidney, the mineralocorticoid and antidiuretic hormones, and the baroreceptors of the carotid sinus and aortic arch are involved in maintaining this equilibrium. Increases or decreases in extracellular fluid volume are directly related to increases or decreases in salt intake and content of the fluid and to increases and decreases in blood pressure levels.

Several lines of evidence suggest that salt may play a role in the initiation or maintenace of hypertension. In man the hypotensive effect of chlorothiazide—which lowers extracellular fluid volume—are undone by a high-salt diet. The addition of salt to the diet of untreated hypertensive patients raises their blood pressure to even higher levels (McDonough and Wilhelmj, 1954). The ingestion of salt by hypertensive persons who previously responded to its dietary restriction by a lowering of blood pressure levels reestablishes their previous high levels (Dole et al., 1951). Salt and water ingestion may cause an increase in the extracellular fluid volume. Hypertensive patients are particularly sensitive to such an increase and respond by a further increase in blood pressure.

The riddle of the pathogenesis of essential hypertension would easily be solved if salt intake were the only causative factor. Actually, salt may contribute to the initiation of, may sustain or enhance preexisting high blood pressure levels, but does not alone seem to cause them, except in certain strains of rats who are sensitive to salt (Ball and Meneely, 1957; Dahl et al., 1960; Meneely et al., 1953, 1954). In other strains of rats, salt must be combined with desoxycorticosterone acetate to produce high blood pressure (Fukuda, 1951; Grollman et al., 1960; Knowlton et al., 1947; Lenel et al., 1948; Sapirstein et al., 1950; Selye et al., 1943). Once the combination of desoxycorticosterone acetate and salt have produced high blood pressure levels, stopping their administration will cause the blood pressure to become normal again. Later, salt by itself will raise the levels. The combined regimen sensitizes some rats to respond only to salt. Therefore, the factors that initiate high blood pressure levels in these rats may be different than those that cause rats later to respond with hypertension to salt alone.

Some epidemiological studies of the incidence and prevalence of essential hypertension implicate salt. In some human populations a linear correlation exists between salt intake and the incidence of hypertension. If the intake of salt is low in a social group, the incidence of hypertension is lower than in another group whose members consume large amounts of salt (Dahl, 1957, 1958, 1960). The amount of salt in a diet is also partly a function of cultural habits. Yet in some individuals, an appetite for salt, independent of cultural habits or the body's requirement for it, seems to exist. Little is known about the variables responsible for the individual craving for salt (Dahl, 1960).

64

The amount of dietary salt, specifically the amount of sodium ion (Gross, 1960), usually determines the amount of renin extractable from the kidney (Gross and Sulser, 1956; Gross and Lichtlen, 1958). In some hypertensive patients, however, plasma renin activity or aldosterone secretion rates are not responsive to salt intake (Luetscher et al., 1969; Streeten et al., 1969; Williams et al., 1970).

The more salt there is in a diet, the greater is the extracellular fluid volume. As the extracellular fluid volume increases, the more renin activity can be detected in serum and the less renin is contained in the kidney. However, the increase in levels of blood sodium do not parallel the increase in blood pressure (Gross, 1960). A variety of regulatory adjustments occur to the increases in serum sodium and renin activity. The arterial pressure at first increases due to an increased cardiac output and stroke volume. Initially there is a fall in peripheral resistance that is then followed by a sustained increase (Coleman and Guyton, 1969).

Any increase of salt in the body increases the extracellular fluid volume to which the circulation adjusts. These adjustments are carried out not only by increases in cardiac output, but by the kidney, by changes in the levels of the mineralocorticoids of the adrenal cortex, and by inhibition of antidiuretic hormone secretion. The kidney responds to an increase in the extracellular fluid volume by increasing urine output in order to reduce the excess of salt and water. In nephrectomized, dialyzed patients, who cannot excrete urine, the blood pressure level fluctuates with changes in the extracellular fluid volume. When the fluid volume increases, the peripheral resistance also does, especially in nephrectomized patients who were previously hypertensive (Muirhead et al., 1966, 1970).

When increases in extracellular fluid volume occur, the level of the blood pressure is determined by a number of additional factors. Epinephrine and angiotensin II are more effective in raising the blood pressure when the blood volume is increased than when it is not. In women with a family history of essential hypertension, the blood pressure is raised by the oral contraceptive pill, which raises levels of plasma angiotensinogen, angiotensin II, and the extracellular fluid volume.

These observations are relevant to an understanding of the nature of the basic physiological defect in essential hypertension. Tobian (1960, 1961, 1972) has suggested that the circulation behaves *as if* there were an excess of extracellular fluid volume (Tobian, 1961) even though the average volume in hypertension may be 10 to 12 percent less than in normotensive persons (Rochlin et al., 1959). He suggests that all the compensatory mechanisms that have been described when the extracellular fluid volume is increased operate upon a normal or below-normal extracellular fluid volume. His suggestion touches upon a central thesis in this chapter that essential hypertension is a "disease of regulation," and that the regulatory disturbances are multiple.

Tobian (1961) has also suggested that an elevated renal arterial pressure in essential hypertension could distend the stretch receptors in the arterial wall and stimulate the juxtaglomerular cells in the wall of the afferent glomerular arteriole. The cells react as if there were an overabundance of extracellular fluid. A further increase in extracellular fluid volume produces an exaggerated sodium diuresis that occurs when sodium, water, or angiotensin are infused into hypertensive patients.

A somewhat different regulatory disturbance in essential hypertension has been suggested by Wilson (1961). According to his view the relationship between the tone of blood vessels and extracellular fluid volume is altered in essential hypertension. The blood-vessel tone in the hypertensive patient is exaggerated for a given fluid volume. Even when the fluid volume is normal, the tone acts as if the fluid volume were increased.

High blood pressure levels can, however, be produced experimentally in animals even when the amount of salt in their diets is low. Presumably the extracellular fluid volume is

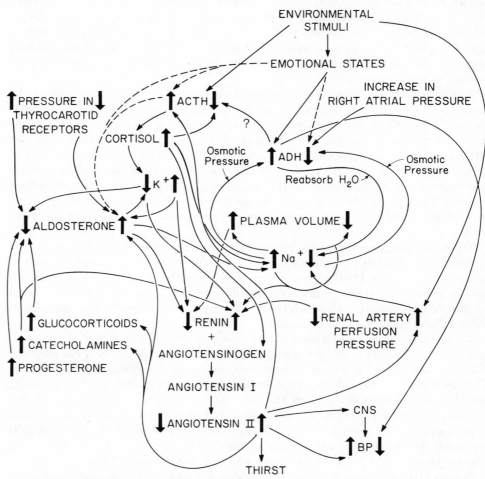

FIGURE 1 The relationships, including feedback regulatory mechanisms, of some of the main mechanisms involved in the maintenance of blood pressure, which have also been implicated in the pathogenesis of essential hypertension. The vertical arrows indicate increases (↑) or decreases (↓) of levels: for example, an increase (↑) of angiotensin II levels in the blood is reflected in increased secretion of aldosterone (↑) and vice versa. The other arrows (→) depict both the positive (as in the foregoing example) and negative feedback regulatory mechanisms involved in the control of blood pressure: other mechanisms are not displayed.

66

also low in salt-restricted animals with a high blood pressure produced by renal artery constriction (Redleaf and Tobian, 1958b).

The regulatory disturbances in essential hypertension suggested by Tobian and Wilson may follow rather than precede the development of high blood pressure. The sodium ion may not initially exert its effect by increasing the extracellular fluid. Large amounts of dietary sodium may also deplete the kidney of its antihypertensive substances such as the prostaglandins.

Large amounts of salt fed to weanling rats for seven weeks, followed by a normal amount of salt in the diet, produces hypertension and reduces the cytoplasmic granules in the renal papilla (Tobian et al., 1969b). The blood pressure of these rats can be reduced by implanting the renal papilla that contains prostaglandins from normotensive rats. In severe human hypertension the papillary granules are also much fewer (Tobian, 1972).

The hypertensive patient paradoxically excretes more salt and water when he partakes of them. The amount of sodium in the body is not only determined by the amount ingested in the diet and the amount excreted in the urine. It is also regulated by the renin-angiotensin-aldosterone system. The serum levels of these hormones fluctuate in concert with the state of sodium balance (Brunner et al., 1972). The complex relationships between sodium and these hormones may be disturbed in some forms of essential hypertension. Some patients with a form of hypertension characterized by low levels of plasma renin activity cannot maintain their blood pressure levels and develop postural hypotension on a low-salt diet. They are unable to conserve their fluid volume on a low-salt diet (Weinberger et al., 1968). In other patients, eating salt does not suppress aldosterone secretion rates as it does in normal persons (Leutscher et al., 1969), nor is the rate of renin secretion responsive to salt deprivation (Streeten et al., 1969; Williams et al., 1970). In normotensive persons, renin, angiotensin II, aldosterone levels, and secretory rates rise as sodium levels in the blood fall, and they decline with rising or excessive sodium levels.

In some forms of essential hypertension the regulation of sodium excretion and reabsorption by the kidney under the influence of aldosterone is disturbed. In other forms, renin and, therefore, aldosterone levels are not responsive to changes in sodium—and its reciprocal ion, potassium—levels in the blood. The regulation of sodium and potassium blood levels is carried out by a number of hormones and organ systems (Figure 1).

The Role of the Antidiuretic Hormone (ADH) in Essential Hypertension

Patients with essential hypertension are sensitive to any increase in extracellular fluid volume. Such increases are produced by eating salt and drinking water. Paradoxically, infusions of salt solution or angiotensin, or increasing the extracellular fluid volume by other methods, produce an exaggerated diuresis in patients. The extracellular fluid volume can also be increased by angiotensin I and II because they are powerful stimuli to drinking water. Another regulator of water metabolism is the antidiuretic hormone (ADH) released by the posterior portion of the pituitary gland, which is under the control of the hypothalamus. Despite reports that the rate of excretion of ADH by the kidney is increased in human and experimental hypertension (Ellis and Grollman, 1949), the role of this important hormone in the disease remains enigmatic. The increased excretion may occur in response to changes in extracellular fluid volume (Sapirstein, 1957) and is, therefore, a secondary phenomenon that would help to sustain high blood pressure levels. ADH and aldosterone are the main but not the only hormones that regulate water and salt metabolism. ADH and aldosterone produce an expansion of the body fluid compartments and increase the glomerular filtration rate. The reabsorption of sodium and chloride is mainly under the influence of aldosterone through a cation exchange mechanism. ADH increases the permeability of the distal convoluted tubules and collecting ducts of the kidney so that water is reabsorbed.

The secretion of ADH is stimulated by an increase in the osmotic pressure of extracellular fluid. ADH, by increasing the reabsorption of water by the kidney, dilutes the extracellular fluid and reduces its osmotic pressure. When the osmolality of extracellular fluid is decreased, ADH secretion is inhibited, and more water is excreted by the kidney. The release of ADH and its inhibition are mediated through the paraventricular nucleus of the hypothalamus, the supraopticohypophyseal tract, and the posterior pituitary gland. When the osmotic pressure of the blood increases, neurons in the supraoptic nucleus of the hypothalamus are excited, and ADH is released from the gland (Brooks et al., 1962; Cross and Green, 1959; Kandel, 1964; Verney, 1947). Stimulating the supraopticohypophyseal tract in rabbits causes ADH secretion and inhibts the excretion of water by the kidney. Water intake is increased by electrical stimulation or the injection of very small volumes of hypertonic saline into the hypothalamus of goats (Andersson and McCann, 1955).

In addition to changes in the osmolality of the blood, various physiological, pharmacological, and psychological factors influence the rate with which ADH is secreted (Rydin and Verney, 1938). Painful stimuli (Mirsky et al., 1954), avoidance conditioning (Mason et al., 1968), and hemorrhage reduce urine excretion, presumably by stimulating ADH secretion. Emotional inhibition of water excretion is also mediated by ADH (Abrahams and Pickford, 1956; Mirsky et al., 1954; O'Connor and Verney, 1945; Verney, 1947). "Stressful" stimuli also release both ACTH and ADH, probably by separate mechanisms (Guillemin et al., 1957; McDonald et al., 1957; Nagareda and Gaunt, 1951; Saffran et al., 1955). The release of ADH is also controlled by the mechanoreceptors in the aorta, carotid arteries, and atrium of the heart. Negative-pressure breathing in the presence of the intact vagus nerve produces a diuresis, presumably through the participation and decreased stimulation of the mechanoreceptors in the left atrium of the heart and the inhibition of ADH secretion (Gauer and Henry, 1963). ADH release is produced by lowering the pressure in the carotid sinus. As the pressure falls, blood volume would be maintained by inhibiting the excretion of water (Perlmutt, 1963; Share and Levy, 1962; Usami et al., 1962). The pathway from the carotid sinus mediating this effect is through the brain.

Some of the central nervous system pathways mediating painful or stressful stimuli and producing ADH release have been mapped by brain-stimulation experiments. ADH release is produced by stimulating the medial midbrain reticular formulation and the interpeduncular nucleus (Hayward and Smith, 1962; Kogel and Rothballer, 1962; Mills and Wang, 1963; Rothballer, 1966). These midbrain sites are capable of phasically increasing neuronal activity in the supraopticohypophyseal system. The release of ADH is brought about by stimulation of midbrain structures and is inhibited by raising the pressure within the carotid sinus, which increases baroreceptor discharge (Rothballer, 1966). Therefore, midbrain structures may integrate ascending neuronal activity from the medulla with activity in the midbrain. Painful peripheral stimuli release ADH. They are mediated by the spinothalamic and spinoreticular tracts and the lateral reticular formation of the medulla oblongata to release ADH. Painful, emotional, and stressful stimuli and changes in blood pressure all effect ADH release and the extracellular fluid volume. Therefore, stressful stimuli may play a role in affecting blood pressure levels in essential hypertension through this mechanism.

The Role of the Adrenal Gland in Essential Hypertension and High Blood Pressure: The Role of Adrenocortical Steroids

ADRENOCORTICAL DISEASE AND HIGH BLOOD PRESSURE

The source of aldosterone is the adrenal cortex. Knowledge of the adrenal gland is central to the understanding of the pathophysiology of essential hypertension. Its weight increases as hypertensive disease progresses (Cooper et al., 1958). In patients with severe hypertension, nodular hyperplasia of the adrenal cortex occurs (Russi et al., 1945; Shamma et al., 1958). The hyperplasia is a compensatory response to the disease and is not due to a primary hyperplasia seen in Conn's syndrome. The secondary form of hyperplasia may be the result of long-standing essential hypertension (Baer et al., 1970). Secondary hyperplasia may be associated with secondary aldosteronism, which can be difficult to distinguish clinically from Conn's syndrome (Conn, 1955, 1961). The relationship of high blood pressure levels to diseases of the adrenal cortex is complex. In Cushing's syndrome due to hyperplasia or adenomata of the adrenal cortex, the increased levels of blood pressure are ascribed to an increased production of hydrocortisone (Christy and Laragh, 1961) or of desoxycorticosterone by the gland (Crane and Harris, 1966). Therefore, high blood pressure levels can occur when one of several adrenocortical hormones are produced in excess.

ACTION OF ALDOSTERONE

Aldosterone, a mineralocorticoid, acts upon the distal tubules of the kidney and causes them to retain sodium and chloride ions and to excrete potassium ions. Aldosterone production and secretion is enhanced in Conn's syndrome, in the malignant phase of essential hypertension, in advanced unilateral renal disease with hypertension, in states in which chronic potassium loss with alkalosis occurs, and in the nephrotic or cirrhotic syndromes with edema. In these pathological states, salt administration does not lower aldosterone secretion as it normally does.

CONTROL OF ALDOSTERONE SECRETION

Angiotensin II is the main, but not the only, regulator of aldosterone production and secretion (Conn et al., 1965; Davis et al., 1962; Mulrow et al., 1962). Its secretion is also influenced by changes in sodium and potassium levels in the blood. Elevated potassium levels and low sodium levels increase aldosterone production but decrease renin secretion

69

(Cannon et al., 1966; Laragh and Stoerk, 1957; Ledingham et al., 1967). Conversely, reduced postassium levels in the serum correlate with reduced aldosterone blood levels (Cannon et al., 1966). Even very small changes in potassium levels produce changes in aldosterone secretion (Boyd and Mulrow, 1972). These changes are independent of the amount of angiotensin II in the blood. In fact, increased levels of serum potassium suppress plasma renin activity but they stimulate aldosterone secretion (Brunner et al., 1970). The effects of potassium on aldosterone secretion are independent of serum sodium levels. The sodium ion also indirectly affects aldosterone production and secretion. Sodium deprivation increases the secretion and renal disposition of aldosterone without measurably changing the concentration of sodium in blood plasma (Luetscher and Axelrad, 1954; Ulick et al., 1958). Changes in the fluid volume of the blood are inversely related to aldosterone excretion (Bartter et al., 1959, 1960). Aldosterone production and changes in the activity of the renin-angiotensin system are brought about by changes in the effective plasma volume (Jose et al., 1970)—and indirectly rather than directly by changes in levels of serum sodium (Bartter et al., 1959; Conn et al., 1965; Cope et al, 1961; Farrell, 1958; Muller et al., 1958; Murlow et al., 1962).

Aldosterone production is also regulated by the nervous system. Stimulation by an increased pulse pressure acting upon the mechanoreceptors at the junction of the thyroid and carotid arteries of the dog, reflexly inhibits aldersterone secretion. A fall in pulse pressure stimulates aldosterone secretion (Bartter et al., 1960). Afferent fibers of the vagus nerve mediate the effect on aldosterone secretion. (The efferent arc of the reflex control of aldosterone secretion is not known.) Increases in venous or right atrial pressure may also reflexly increase aldosterone secretion. The reflex is abolished by nephrectomy but not by denervation of the adrenal glands (Carpenter et al., 1961; Davis et al., 1960).

ACTH also has a transient stimulating effect on aldosterone secretion (Davis et al., 1970; Laragh, 1961), although aldosterone secretion is not altered very much by hypophysectomy. Therefore, the pituitary control of aldosterone secretion has not been firmly established, but is actively being investigated at the moment. The pineal gland has also been implicated in the regulation of aldosterone secretion (Yankopolous et al., 1959). Farrell (1959a, b) claimed that the pineal gland secretes a hormone that enhances aldosterone secretion. Later he claimed that another pineal factor inhibits the secretion of ACTH. He believed that the pineal gland produced two factors that could alter aldosterone secretion. This was confirmed by Wurtman et al. (1959) who found that pinealectomy was followed by adrenal hypertrophy. Juan (1963) showed that ACTH secretion increases after removal of the pineal gland. Pineal extracts, by inhibiting β-hydroxylation in the adrenal cortex, could reduce the production of aldosterone, cortisol, corticosterone, and cortisone (Mess, 1967). The concept that the pineal gland is involved in the regulation of aldosterone production has been challenged (Barbour et al., 1965; Davis, 1961; Denton, 1961; Wurtman et al., 1960).

In summary, aldosterone is regulated by angiotensin, the content of the potassium ion in blood serum, the extracellular fluid volume, and probably by increased blood pressure levels acting through mechanoreceptors in the arteries of the neck. It may also be under the control of the pituitary and pineal glands. Because aldosterone is intimately concerned with regulating the sodium and potassium content of body fluids, it is central to our understanding of blood pressure control. Excessive aldosterone secretion raises the blood pressure. Although increases of aldosterone secretion usually only occur in the advanced or malignant phases of hypertensive vascular disease, several lines of evidence suggest that in some subgroups of patients with essential hypertension the regulation of aldosterone secretion is disturbed. In other subgroups the rate of its metabolic disposition is retarded.

THE ROLE OF ALDOSTERONE IN ESSENTIAL HYPERTENSION

Angiotensin II consistently stimulates the secretion of aldosterone and, therefore, the retention in the body of salt and water. The renin-angiotensin-aldosterone mechanism is believed to play a part in initiating essential hypertension. Two lines of evidence argue against this hypothesis because increases in aldosterone secretion and excretion probably only occur in malignant or advanced cases of hypertension (Garst et al., 1960; Genest, 1961; Laragh et al., 1960), and are secondary to increased levels of renin and angiotensin II (Biron et al., 1961). In normal persons or patients with the normal or high-renin forms of hypertension, urinary aldosterone excretion is highly correlated with plasma renin levels (Laragh et al., 1972). However, there are instances of low-renin hypertension that are associated with deviations in the normal mechanisms regulating the interactions between renin, angiotensin II, and aldosterone. In the presence of low plasma renin (and presumably of low angiotensin II) activity, urinary aldosterone excretion can be low, normal, or high.

In low-renin hypertension considerable variation in the responses of renin and aldosterone levels to changes in sodium balance occur. In some instances renin levels vary with changes in sodium balance, but aldosterone excretion levels do not change; they remain high and fixed. In other instances, changes in sodium balance do not affect low plasma renin levels but do alter aldosterone excretion. In a fourth group of low renin hypertensive patients, renin and aldosterone levels increase with a fall in sodium levels (Laragh et al., 1972). It has been suggested that the variations from the normal in low-renin hypertension are due to different disturbances in the usual feedback regulation of renin, aldosterone, and fluid volume (see Figure 2). When aldosterone levels are high and fixed, idiopathic bilateral adrenal hyperplasia may occur, despite normal potassium levels (Baer et al., 1970). Patients with a baseline of low renin levels and normal-to-high aldosterone excretion, which both respond to changes in sodium balance, have an increased sensitivity or responsiveness of the adrenal cortex to angiotensin II (Laragh et al., 1972). When low renin and low aldosterone levels occur in hypertensive patients, both responsive to shifts in sodium balance and fluid volume, the vasoconstrictive properties of angiotensin II (acting either on the brain stem or directly on blood vessels) may be enhanced. Alternatively, such patients may have a renal defect that produces an excessive reabsorption of salt in the presence of low aldosterone levels (Lowenstein et al., 1970). As a consequence, an abnormal expansion of plasma and extracellular fluid volume occurs (Jose et al., 1970).

Another explanation for the role of aldosterone in the pathophysiology of essential hypertension has been put forward by Genest (1974). Circulating levels of plasma aldosterone fall into the high-normal range in about one-third of patients with benign essential hypertension. They are somewhat raised, not because the production or secretion

71

rates of aldosterone are high but because its metabolic clearance rates are lower than normal. These investigators suggest that a hepatic defect occurs in patients who have normal or low plasma renin levels and, therefore, should have normal or undetectable aldosterone levels. The abnormally low clearance rate of the mineralocorticoid may be due to a decreased hepatic blood flow that, in turn, may either reduce the chemical inactivation of aldosterone in the liver or increase its globulin-binding in plasma.

No one has proven that disturbances in aldosterone metabolism or its regulating mechanisms antecede the development of essential hypertension. But these new data suggest that patients with essential hypertension fall into several subgroups. Therefore, no single mechanism could account for the pathophysiology of all the subgroups of essential hypertension.

THE ADRENAL CORTICOIDS: CORTISOL AND DESOXYCORTICOSTERONE

The several glucocorticoids of the adrenal cortex play an enigmatic role in the pathogenesis of essential hypertension. One of the adrenal glucocorticoids that can produce elevated levels of blood pressure in animals is desoxycorticosterone. The mode of action of the glucocorticoids in essential hypertension is complex; they interact with and modify the action of aldosterone. They prevent prostaglandin release (Lewis and Piper, 1975). Aldosterone produces elevated blood pressure in patients treated for adrenal cortical insufficiency with glucocorticoids. In these patients the elevated blood pressure produced by aldosterone is associated with sodium retention, which is attenuated by cortisol and corticosterone (Leutscher et al., 1954, 1969, 1973; Ross et al., 1960). The production and secretion of the glucocorticoids is regulated by ACTH, which also produces acute increases in aldosterone secretion (Davis et al., 1970). If ACTH is administered for a prolonged time, aldosterone secretion either returns to normal or to subnormal levels (Newton and Laragh, 1968a) probably because of the associated increase of glucocorticoid secretion that reduces aldosterone production and secretion (Newton and Laragh, 1968b). Normally, the glucocorticoids appear to maintain vascular reactivity and the pressor response to norepinephrine (Fritz and Levine, 1951; Ramey et al., 1951). But in hypertensive patients glucocorticoids do not increase vascular reactivity to vasoconstrictors such as norepinephrine. Aldosterone and salt alter vascular reactivity instead (Mendlowitz, 1967) by increasing the water and salt content of the arteriolar wall and, hence, its elasticity (Knowlton, 1960; Laramore and Grollman, 1950; Tobian et al., 1961, 1969). The changes in vascular reactivity to norepinephrine in essential hypertension help to sustain elevated blood pressure levels but do not initiate them (Grollmam, 1960). Changes in serum levels of the glucocorticoids are the consequences of the advanced stages of hypertensive disease. In less-advanced hypertension, the *in vitro* synthesis of corticosterone in the adrenal glands is enhanced. In severe hypertensive disease, cortisol synthesis is depressed. Cortisol output in the adrenal vein, measured at the time of operation, is lower when diastolic blood pressure is higher (Cooper et al., 1958). Increases in plasma or urinary cortisol, cortisone, tetrahydrocortisone, or 17-hydroxycorticosteroids in essential hypertension occur in some patients or some forms of the disease (Genest et al., 1960; Vermeulen and Van der Straeten, 1963). Urinary

72

pregnanetriol, or the ratio of pregnanetriol to aldosterone, is depressed in essential, renal, or malignant hypertension (Genest et al., 1960; Vermeulen and Van der Straeten, 1963). Progesterone inhibits the sodium-retaining effect of aldosterone (Genest et al., 1960), as do other glucocorticoids, and both Genest et al. (1960) and Armstong (1959) have found that progesterone lowers the blood pressure of hypertensive patients, possibly by its effect on aldosterone levels.

In a series of patients with labile essential hypertension who were on a controlled diet of salt, 45 percent had progesterone levels three times higher than normal (Genest, 1974). When sodium intake is restricted, progesterone levels usually rise in normal subjects. In patients with high progesterone levels the increase is much less. Thus, there may be an inability to increase progesterone levels in these patients when their aldosterone levels are increased on a low-sodium diet. Therefore, in some patients with labile essential hypertension, another regulatory disturbance exists consisting of a diminished progesterone response to a low-salt diet. In the presence of this regulatory disturbance, the blood pressure would not fall as completely on a low-salt diet as it should.

A complete account of all the hormonal factors involved in blood pressure regulation and in essential hypertension has not yet been rendered: but the interactions of the hormones in the normal and diseased state are multiple and complex.

The mineralocorticoid desoxycorticosterone has potent hypertensive properties only in the presence of salt. On a diet poor in salt, large doses of desoxycorticosterone acetate produce modest elevations of blood pressure in the rat (Grollman et al., 1940; Knowlton et al., 1947; Selye et al., 1943). When rats drink a 1 percent salt solution the same dose of desoxycorticosterone acetate produces much greater elevations of blood pressure. The blood pressure remains high as long as the rats continue to drink saline. If the rat drinks ordinary drinking water instead of saline, the blood pressure falls. Gross (1956, 1960) and Gross and Lichtlen (1958) showed that the renin content of the kidney is directly proportional to the amounts of salt and water the rat ingests. If the salt intake is high, renin is released from the kidney in these rats.

Once excessive salt and desoxycorticosterone acetate have produced an elevated blood pressure and they are discountinued, the blood pressure falls to normal. But these rats remain permanently sensitive to excessive salt intake. They develop a high blood pressure when they again eat salt in excess. The rat is the only animal that develops high blood pressure when fed excessive amounts of salt after desoxycorticosterone acetate injections. The rabbit and the dog do not.

Desoxycorticosterone-salt hypertension in rats is associated with an increase in the activity of peripheral sympathetic nerves and of the adrenal medulla (De Champlain, 1972; De Champlain and Van Amerigen, 1973). While peripheral sympathetic activity increases, a decrease in norepinephrine turnover rates in the medulla oblongata occurs (De Champlain and van Amerigen, 1973; Nakamura et al., 1971). Sympathetic ganglionic blocking agents lower the blood pressure of pretreated rats but do not increase norepinephrine turnover rates in the medulla oblongata. The lowered turnover rates in the medulla are related to the increased peripheral sympathetic activity. If noradrenergic neurons in the medulla oblongata are destroyed by the prior intraventicular installation of 6-hydroxydopamine, high blood pressure levels and the increased peripheral sympathetic activity are prevented from occurring in treated rats (Finch et al., 1972). Once high blood pressure levels are established in these rats, 6-hydroxydopamine treatment does not lower them (Finch et al., 1972; Haeusler et al., 1972b).

Desoxycorticosterone-salt hypertension in rats is, therefore, mediated through the brain stem. The treatment with salt and desoxycorticosterone acetate lowers norepinephrine turnover rates. As noradrenergic activity in the medulla oblongata diminishes, peripheral sympathetic activity increases. Presumably, there are noradrenergic neurons in the brain stem that usually inhibit vasoconstrictor discharge down the spinal cord. In this form of experimental hypertension, the neurons are less-active and disinhibition occurs. Once high blood pressure levels are installed, some other mechanisms sustain them, because destruction of noradrenergic neurons in the medulla oblongata only prevents its development but does not "cure it."

The increased peripheral sympathetic activity is well-documented in this form of experimental hypertension. The increase should be accompanied by increases of blood levels of the enzyme DBH. But it is not. The elevated blood-pressure levels produced in rats by treatment with desoxycorticosterone acetate and salt actually results in a fall of serum DBH levels (Williams et al., 1972b). The repeated immobilization of rats also produces high blood pressure levels. In restrained rats the catecholamine synthesizing enzyme DBH is increased. Therefore, the conclusion is justified that different experimental techniques produce high blood pressure levels in rats by different mechanisms. Yet the same techniques may produce high blood pressure levels in one animal genus but not in another.

OTHER MINERALOCORTICOIDS: THE ROLE OF 18-HYDROXY-DESOXYCORTICOSTERONE

Low-renin essential hypertension in man may be produced by the excessive production of another corticosteroid, 18-hydroxy-desoxycorticosterone (18-OH desoxycorticosterone) (Gross, 1971); 18-OH desoxycorticosterone is a mineralocorticoid that suppresses renin, aldosterone, and serum potassium levels, thereby causing salt and water retention. It is regulated by ACTH in man and in rat.

The administration of 18-OH desoxycorticosterone to unilaterally nephrectomized rats significantly increases the blood pressure to high levels (Oliver et al., 1973). Usually, it takes 16 days of the administration of 18-OH desoxycorticosterone for the blood pressure to increase in nephrectomized rats. But in the salt-sensitive strain of rats, no nephrectomy is required and 18-OH desoxycorticosterone plays a significant and etiologic role in elevating the blood pressure. In human hypertension the role of 18-OH desoxycorticosterone needs further clarification. It may play a pathogenetic but not an etiologic role in some forms of human essential hypertension. In other patients it may sustain high blood pressure levels.

THE ROLE OF THE CATECHOLAMINES IN ESSENTIAL HYPERTENSION

The central and peripheral sympathetic nervous system and the catecholamines have a wide variety of actions on the heart, the kidney, and the arterioles. Increased peripheral sympathetic activity may increase the heart rate, the force of the heart beat, and cardiac output, contract arterioles to raise the peripheral resistance, and release renin (Davis, 1974). Central catecholaminergic and serotonergic neurons are involved in the control of the circulation and blood pressure (Chalmers, 1975). Central catecholaminergic mechanisms have been implicated in the initiation of several different forms of experimental high blood pressure in animals.

Nonetheless the role of the sympathetic nervous system and its neurotransmitters in the etiology and pathogenesis of essential hypertension are not fully understood. Several competing hypotheses that could account for the increase in peripheral resistance exist. One hypothesis proposes that increased tonic sympathetic vasoconstrictor activity leads to the increased release of norepinephrine within the arteriolar wall. Normally, norepinephrine produces only vasoconstriction in the skin, muscle, and intestinal blood vessels (Folkow and Uvnäs, 1948; Folkow et al., 1965; Youmans et al., 1955). The walls of these blood vessels contain only norepinephrine (Schmiterlow, 1948).

Another hypothesis states that there is a heightened sensitivity of the arterioles to normal tonic sympathetic activity. A third hypothesis holds that once hypertrophy of the arteriolar wall encroaches on its lumen, regular changes in sympathetic discharge produce an unusual increase in the resistance to blood flow (Folkow, 1952, 1971; Folkow et al., 1956). According to the last two hypotheses, sympathetic discharge and the release of neurotransmitter substances, either from the adrenal medulla or from the site of innervation of the arterioles, is normal, but the response of the arteriole is altered. The test of this alternative hypothesis is difficult and cannot be carried out merely by studying increased blood or urinary excretion levels of catecholamines.

Some investigators have found increase of catecholamine levels in essential hypertension early in its course (Engelman et al., 1970; Goodall and Bogdonoff, 1961; Holtz et al., 1947; von Euler et al., 1954) or only in the malignant phase of the disease (Goldenberg et al., 1948). Most investigators have found normal levels in every phase of the disease.

These contradictory results can partly be explained by the presence or absence of impaired kidney function. In hypertensive patients with normal kidney function, catecholamine excretion is increased. Impaired kidney function reduces catecholamine excretion (Ikoma, 1965).

That the catecholamines play a partial role either in the etiology, pathogenesis, or pathophysiology of essential hypertension is attested to by the fact that reserpine, monoamine oxidase inhibitors and a number of other drugs that affect catecholamine metabolism reduce the blood pressure in hypertensive patients (DiPalma, 1961). Reserpine is believed to produce its hypotensive effect mainly by depleting peripheral neuroeffector sites and sympathetic ganglia of their stores of catecholamines (Costa, 1961; Holzbauer and Vogt, 1956). Drugs that do not deplete peripheral norepinephrine stores do not lower the blood pressure. Guanethidine causes a fall in blood pressure by reducing the stores of norepinephrine at peripheral synapses. But reserpine also depletes the brain of serotonin and of the catecholamines. The hypotensive action of reserpine is probably partly mediated through its central, not only its peripheral, actions. Reserpine also lowers epinephrine and norepinephrine levels in the adrenal medulla (Kroneberg and Schümann, 1959). Reserpine given to cats and dogs causes a slow and progressive decline in efferent splanchnic nerve activity and a fall in blood pressure. The effect of reserpine on blood pressure is different from that produced by tetraethylammonium chloride and mecamylamine, which act peripherally (McCubbin and Page, 1958). Some drugs that are effective in the treatment of human essential hypertension may act only peripherally, while others act both centrally and peripherally to reduce sympathetic activity.

Much remains to be learned: in animals the same drugs may increase or have no effects on blood pressure levels (Brodie and Costa, 1961; Franco-Browder et al., 1958). The fact that these drugs lower the blood pressure in humans suggests that the sympathetic nervous system plays some role—perhaps only a sustaining one—in essential hypertension.

Conversely, a genetic and predisposing defect may be present in the form of the altered synthesis, storage or disposition of the catecholamines. De Champlain et al. (1969) have suggested that this defect consists of a reduced capacity of the storage granules in sympathetic nerve endings to bind and store norepinephrine. In rats made hypertensive by pretreatment with desoxycorticosterone acetate and salt, an inverse relationship exists between the systolic blood pressure and the capacity of the heart to store norepinephrine. As a result of a failure to store it, larger amounts of free norepinephrine are physiologically active in these animals. The increased liberation of norepinephrine precedes the increase in blood pressure in these animals.

The increased turnover of norepinephrine has been described in experimental neurogenic hypertension in various species of animals, in rats of the spontaneously hypertensive strain (Louis et al., 1968), and in rats made hypertensive by encapsulating one kidney and removing the other (Volicer et al., 1968). Impaired storage of the catecholamines in hypertensive human subjects has also been described (Gitlow et al., 1964) and may explain the reports of increased excretion of the catecholamines if the kidney functions normally (Stott and Robinson, 1967).

Once released, the catecholamines may play another role in essential hypertension by their effects on electrolyte metabolism and the kidney. Small or intermediate doses of injected norepinephrine increase urine flow, presumably by reducing ADH secretion (Pickford, 1952). When norepinephrine is given in larger doses, glomerular filtration rate and urine volume are diminished (Handley and Moyer, 1954; King and Baldwin, 1956). The reduction of filtration rate is always accompanied by a reduction in the excretion of sodium and potassium (King and Baldwin, 1956; McSmythe et al., 1952; Mills et al., 1953). In normal subjects infusion of a saline solution after sympathetic transmission is blocked with guanethidine increases the excretion of sodium and usually enhances the glomerular filtration rate. If, in addition to sodium and guanethidine, a mineralocorticoid is injected, the excretion of sodium is still increased (Gill et al., 1964). Therefore, the catecholamines play a complex role in the regulation of electrolyte metabolism and modify the effects of corticosteroids.

In patients with labile, borderline hypertension, an increased β-adrenergic drive on the heart raises the cardiac output. When lying down, these patients excrete more than the usual amounts of epinephrine and norepinephrine in the urine. When these patients sit up their norepinephrine levels rise further and excessively, their epinephrine levels fall slightly, their dopamine levels fall less than expected, and their plasma renin activity increase more than in normotensive persons. On a low-sodium diet the differences between borderline hypertensive patients and normotensive subjects disappear.

Therefore, in labile, borderline essential hypertension there seems to be excessive adrenergic activity and mildly increased plasma renin levels (Frohlich et al., 1970), in contrast with normal and other forms of essential hypertension, which have stable, elevated blood pressure levels and normal cardiac output. In patients with borderline hypertension isoproterenol produces a greater and more persistent increase in renin activity (Genest, 1974) that is blocked by propranolol (Hamet et al., 1973a, b).

In labile, borderline hypertension the sympathetic nervous system exerts its effects by increasing renin activity, cardiac output and heart rate, sodium retention, and a positive sodium balance. In these patients, increases in peripheral vascular resistance eventually occur, and other and sustaining mechanisms take over to produce more-stable elevated blood pressure levels with a normal cardiac output.

The cause of the increased sympathetic nervous system activity early in borderline hypertension is unknown. In this form of hypertension the sympathetic nervous system probably plays a primary, initiating role. But we do not know whether the increased sympathetic activity is central or peripheral in origin. If it could be shown that the increased sympathetic nervous system is central in origin, the neurogenic theory of some, if not all forms of essential hypertension would receive some support. In the meantime, patients with borderline and labile essential hypertension should be studied socially and psychologically in order to try to account for their increased sympathetic activity.

The Role of the Central Nervous System in the Control of Blood Pressure and in Essential Hypertension

MULTIFACTOR AND NEUROGENIC THEORIES OF ESSENTIAL HYPERTENSION

The neurogenic theory of the etiology and pathogenesis of essential hypertension is currently not popular. In its original form it placed the entire burden for the etiology of the disease on the central nervous system and its autonomic and neuroendocrine outflow tracts. The neurogenic theory has been replaced by multifactor theories of etiology, the best known of which is Page's mosaic theory (1960). Multifactor hypotheses are favored by many besides Page (Peterson, 1963; Pickering, 1961; Shapiro, 1973). These theorists contend that linear, single-cause, explanatory theories do not adequately cover the clinical facts. They contend that there are many regulatory mechanisms in equilibrium that control tissue perfusion and blood pressure. Some of these mechanisms are chemical; others are neural and cardiovascular: they regulate cardiac output, blood volume and viscosity, electrolyte and water balance, and the caliber, elasticity, and reactivity of blood vessels. Each mechanism in turn influences the other (See Figure 1).

The mosaic or other multifactor theories lack parsimony, but they do account for most of the known facts about the disease. Multifactor theories imply the operation of complex feedback regulatory devices in normal blood pressure control and in essential hypertension. Any one of these regulatory devices may be biased, or may deviate from the norm, in essential hypertension to alter their interrelationships. The multifactor theories do not tell us how these relationships are altered to produce essential hypertension or the exact nature of these alterations: hereditary and congenital factors may produce structural alterations to effect the function of the kidney. For example, these alterations may lie

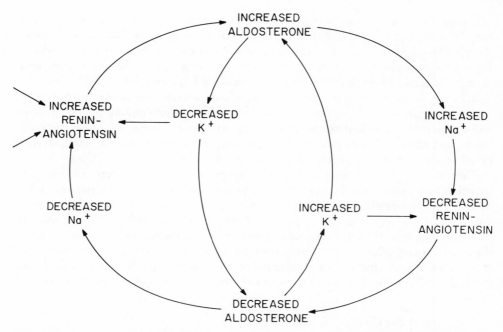

FIGURE 2 **Feedback Regulatory System of the Renin-Angiotensin-Aldosterone System and Its Relationship to Variations in Sodium and Potassium Levels.** The arrows on the left indicate other influences (e.g., dilatation of the renal artery and sympathetic tonic and phasic influences which increase renin secretion and activity). Modified with permission from Laragh et al. in *American J. of Medicine.* Copyright 1972 by Dun-Donnelley.

dormant and blood pressure levels may be normal, until a drug, such as the oral contraceptive pill, elicits the latent tendency.

In women who develop hypertension when taking oral contraceptives, some have family histories of hypertension, or they have congenital fibromuscular hyperplasia of the renal artery that has been "dormant" and only reveals itself in hypertension after the oral contraceptive is taken (Shapiro, 1973). The family history or the congenital renal artery lesion constitute latent tendencies to high blood pressure that are activated by the oral contraceptives. Each one of these factors by itself is insufficient to raise the blood pressure. Not every woman taking the pill develops hypertension.

Most multifactor theories about the nature of essential hypertension emphasize the etiological role of disturbances in autoregulatory mechanisms in the arterioles, in the kidney, or in the regulatory relationship between the kidney and the adrenal gland. Changes in the regulation of these organ systems by the brain are not currently emphasized in etiological or pathogenetic theories of essential or other forms of hypertension. It was once argued that the nervous system could not be involved in the pathogenesis of renal hypertension because renal denervation does not prevent the development of renal hypertension (Page, 1935). The pathogenetic role of the sympathetic nervous system in essential hypertension was also dismissed, because prolonged stimulation of the splanchnic nerves fails to produce self-perpetuating, chronic hypertension in dogs (Kubicek et al., 1953). Until recently no clear-cut evidence existed that excesses or aberrations in pressor catecholamine levels or metabolism contribute to the etiology of any form of essential hypertension (Wilson, 1961; Page and McCubbin, 1965). With the development of new techniques, it has been shown that, at least in some hospitalized patients with essential hypertension, plasma or urinary catecholamine levels are elevated (Engelman et al., 1970; Frohlich et al., 1970).

The most telling argument against the neurogenic hypothesis is the evidence that the kidney is the primary initiating agent of essential hypertension. A normal kidney transplanted into a hypertensive patient will develop the vascular lesions of malignant hypertension unless the diseased kidney is removed (Merrill et al., 1956; Murray et al., 1958). Either the high blood pressure levels or the diseased kidney in some way turns the normal kidney into a diseased one.

In animals, hypertension occurs when both kidneys are removed (Braun-Menendez and von Euler, 1947; Grollman et al., 1949). When a normal kidney is then transplanted into a dog without kidneys, the blood pressure returns to normal levels (Kolff et al., 1954). The high blood pressure in an animal without kidneys seems to depend, in part, on the amounts of sodium and protein in the diet (Orbison et al., 1952; Kolff and Page, 1954) or on increased hydration that presumably causes an increased effective plasma volume (Merrill et al., 1961).

These examples are powerful arguments for the role of the kidney in the pathogenesis of essential hypertension. In the first example, a normal kidney becomes diseased. The inference can be drawn from the second example that the kidney regulates the blood pressure by virtue of its role in maintaining the extracellular fluid volume in an equilibrium condition.

The kidney also contains the antihypertensive prostaglandins; therefore, removing it would deprive the body of these substances. Small wonder that the kidney is often considered to be the main initiator of essential hypertension.

The disease is considered by many to be due to an autoregulatory disturbance within the kidney, specifically an imbalance between its hypertensive and antihypertensive mechanisms. Alternatively, Floyer (1955) has suggested that the kidney maintains a normal blood pressure by inhibiting extrarenal pressor mechanisms. This inhibitory mechanism is impaired either by constriction of a renal artery or a fall in renal artery pressure and the subsequent release of renin. Once impaired, a disinhibition of the extrarenal pressor mechanisms occurs and blood pressure levels rise. The pressor mechanisms are sustained by the brain.

Certainly, congenital and acquired kidney disease produces secondary hypertension. Essential hypertension can also eventuate in kidney disease that sustains high blood pressure levels. The evidence is certainly very strong that the kidney can initiate and sustain high blood pressure levels. Therefore, multifactor theories are unnecessary to explain the pathogensis of essential hypertension.

Nonetheless, strong evidence exists that even when the kidney initiates high blood pressure levels, it does so through the mediation of the brain. The development of high blood pressure in animals, produced by renal artery constriction, can be averted by pretreatment with intraventricular 6-hydroxydopamine that destroys catecholaminergic neurons (Chalmers, 1975). But once high blood pressure levels are established in these animals, 6-hydroxydopamine treatment does not lower the blood pressure (Finch et al., 1972; Lewis et al., 1973). The sequence of events is probably as follows: constricting the renal artery releases renin and angiotensin II is produced. Angiotensin II enters the brain via the area postrema (Joy and Lowe, 1970; Lewis et al., 1973) to produce powerful pressor effects that are in turn mediated by sympathetic discharge (Ferrario et al., 1969, 1972; Fukyama et al., 1973; Gildenberg, 1971; Scroop and Lowe, 1968; Sweet and Brody, 1970). Angiotensin II, when infused in very small amounts intervertebrally, significantly increases the blood pressure. Its effect can be blocked by pretreatment with reserpine (Sweet and Brody, 1971) and by destruction of central catecholaminergic neurons. The sympathetic discharge not only produces vasoconstriction but may release more renin from the kidney (Bunag et al., 1966).

The brain, therefore, appears to participate in the initial rise in blood pressure produced by experimental renal artery constriction. Hypertension can be produced experimentally by many other methods. In these other forms of experimental hypertension, the brain seems to pay a primary initiating, not only a mediating, role.

Hypertension can also be produced by denervation of the baroreceptors (Kezdi, 1967), by conditioning techniques, and by social manipulation. The development of spontaneous hypertension in selected strains of rats can be prevented by the intraventricular injection of 6-hydroxydopamine (Finch et al., 1972). The brain also participates in the development of desoxycorticosterone-salt hypertension in rats. Therefore, the brain is either involved in the initiation or the mediation of the initial phases of experimental hypertension. Because destruction of central catecholaminergic neurons prevents the development of some forms of experimental hypertension but does not "cure" it, one may conclude that a different chain of mechanisms are involved in initiating than in sustaining high blood pressure levels. If this conclusion is correct, the multifactor theory is alos correct.

THE ROLE OF THE CENTRAL NERVOUS SYSTEM IN THE INITIATION OF HYPERTENSION

Central to current psychosomatic theories is that is that social and psychological factors predispose to initiate, sustain, or alter the course of essential hypertension. Some experiments in animals support the idea that social and psychological factors may initiate hypertension, presumably through the brain. Other experiments suggest that the primary initiating role of the kidney is mediated through the brain. Conversely, there is also evidence that the brain can alter the function of the kidney and many other systems that regulate blood pressure levels.

The brain also participates in the regulation of the autonomic nervous system, renal artery flow, ADH output, adrenal corticosteroid, and renin release. It ultimately regulates plasma volume, salt and water metabolism, and the peripheral resistance. The central nervous system is sometimes thought to have no influence in essential hypertension because a direct neural effect on the kidney has not been demonstrated. Yet the nervous system can modify renal function in other ways (Hoff and Green, 1936; Lund, 1943). Psychological stimuli decrease diodrast clearance, increase insulin clearance, and diminish renal plasma flow (Meehan, 1960; Smith, 1939, 1940). Stimulation of the supraorbital gyrus diminishes renal blood flow (Cort, 1953). Hoff et al (1951) produced renocortical ischemia sufficient to produce tubular necrosis by stimulation of the anterior sigmoid gyrus of cats. Stimulation of the dorsal medulla lateral to the midline increases blood pressure and urine volume and diminishes the glomerular filtration rate. Stimulation at the level of the obex increases glomerular filtration rate and urine volume (Wise and Ganong, 1960).

Therefore, the initial impetus to high blood pressure may be imparted by the brain to the kidney, because the brain can lower renal artery blood flow and release renin. Alternatively, the brain may initially act to disinhibit the inhibitory action of the kidney on extrarenal pressor mechanisms. Once the function of the kidney is altered, reflex sympathetic activity may increase (Chalmers, 1975; Reed et al., 1944). In fact, in experimental renal hypertension, there is a decreased hypotensive response to agents blocking the sympathetic ganglia and to attempts to reduce the increased sympathetic vasoconstriction and stimulation of the heart (Henning, 1969; Kezdi, 1962; Kezdi and Wennemark, 1958; Page and McCubbin, 1951; Volicer et al., 1969). Chemical or immunosympathectomy of peripheral sympathetic nerves prevents the development of renal hypertension, especially if chemical sympathectomy is combined with adrenalectomy (Ayitey-Smith and Varma, 1970; De Champlain and van Amerigen, 1973; Finch et al., 1972; Haeusler et al., 1972b). In rabbits, the longer experimental renal hypertension lasts, the less likely is nephrectomy to lower the blood pressure (Pickering, 1945), a result suggesting that renal hypertension is eventually sustained by an extrarenal mechanism.

Destruction of the nervous system by pithing reduces the elevated arterial pressure in experimental renal hypertension, however long-standing. If pithing is carried out while angiotensin is infused, the blood pressure is not reduced, which suggests that angiotensin in sufficient dosage acts directly on the circulation (Dock, 1940; Taquini et al., 1961).

Other experiments have also suggested that a tandem mechanism is involved in the experimental renal hypertension that is produced by interfering with the renal circulation (Drury and Schapiro, 1956; Gomez et al., 1960; Reed et al., 1944). The experiments have indicated that at first a pressor substance is released by the kidney and later an additional (perhaps neural) mechanism is involved in sustaining elevated blood pressure levels.

SOME GENERAL PRINCIPLES: THE DIFFERENTIAL REGULATION OF CARDIOVASCULAR MECHANISMS BY THE BRAIN

Conclusions drawn from studies on the neurogenic control of blood pressure are limited. Much of our knowlege about the regulation of the circulation and the control of blood pressure by the nervous system is derived from observations made on excised organs and anesthetized animals. Only with the development of new recording methods has it become feasible to make observations on intact unanesthetized animals. These new techniques eliminate the various artifacts caused by exposing the heart and lungs in acute experiments and by anesthesia. Behavioral observations can also be made in intact, unanesthetized animals. Behavior and cardiovascular function can be studied together during exercise, while the animal is interacting with its environment, or while brain stimulation is being carried out. Chronic brain stimulation may be used to induce elevations of blood pressure while an animal's behavior is observed.

The rapid cardiovascular adjustments that precede and accompany exercise demonstrate the participation of the brain in the regulation of the circulation. These adjustments were once thought to be instigated solely by peripheral mechanisms. The onset of vasodilation, increased blood flow in muscle, increased heart rate and cardiac output in anticipation and at the start of exercise are produced by the nervous system. They are the autonomic concomitants of the muscular activity of exercise. The cardiovascular changes at the start of exercise can be abolished by lesions in the fields of Forel. They can be reproduced by stimulation in this area in resting animals (Rushmer, 1958). Therefore, integrated patterns of cardiovascular and motor activity on exercise are orchestrated by the brain.

Different cardiovascular changes may be quite specific to a given behavioral state, or activity. In man, integrated patterns of cardiovascular changes occur in emotional states and during mental effort or physical exercise (Barcroft et al., 1960; Blair et al., 1959; Brod, 1959, 1970). In animals, too, quite specific cardiovascular changes occur during different behavioral states, including during states with strong emotional overtones. In preparing to fight another cat, a cat shows bradycardia, a decreased cardiac output, and vasoconstriction in the iliac and mesenteric vessels. When he strikes the other cat, the heart rate and cardiac output increase, the iliac bed dilates, and the mesenteric bed constricts. In neither case does the blood pressure rise very much (Adams et al., 1968).

Theoretically, stimulation at different brain sites should also produce different patterns of changes in the circulation. This occurs in practice. Stimulation of the cerebral cortex facilitates vasomotor discharge and increases the blood pressure. The stimulus is mediated by the pyramidal tract that begins in the sigmoid gyrus and the pericruciate cortex. The pyramidal tract regulates vasomotor activity through collaterals to the pons and medulla (Landau, 1953; Rossi and Brodal, 1956; Wall and Davis, 1951). Stimulating the pyramidal tract electrically raises the blood pressure and produces movements. Other cortical areas may produce their pressor effects by pathways to the hypothalamus, because lesions of the hypothalamus abolish vasomotor responses to stimulation of the surfaces of the posterior orbital gyrus.

On stimulation of frontal and temporal cortex, the blood pressure can be both raised and lowered in many mammals, including man (Anand and Dua, 1956a, b; Kaada et al., 1949; Sachs et al., 1949). Several rhinencephalic areas (the anterior limbic cortex, anterior insula, and the hippocampal gyrus) produce significant changes in blood pressure when stimulated electrically (Kaada, 1951). The cingulate gyrus and the amygdala are also involved in blood pressure regulation (Anand and Dua, 1956a; Kaada, 1951; Pool and Ransohoff, 1949; Ward, 1948). When a number of midline structures—the nonspecific thalamic nuclei and the midbrain reticular system—are subjected to high-frequency electrical stimulation, marked elevations of blood pressure occur. The effects of such stimulation persist after stimulation ceases. Stimulation of the vermis of the cerebellum modifies ongoing activity in bulbopontine, vasomotor, and hypothalamic centers, and can produce either elevation or depression of blood pressure levels (Moruzzi, 1940, 1950; Zanchetti and Zoccolini, 1954).

82

High-frequency stimulation of the hypothalamus produces acute phasic increases in blood pressure (Hess, 1949). The rate of hypothalamic stimulation is linearly related to the discharge frequency in single fibers of the inferior-cardiac and cervical-sympathetic nerves: the higher the rate of hypothalamic stimulation, the greater is the discharge frequency. Hypothalamic stimulation also increases the blood pressure increments produced by stimulation of a peripheral sensory nerve (Pitts et al., 1941, 1941/2). After hypothalamic stimulation is ended, the blood pressure remains elevated for several minutes due to the release of vasopressin or of catecholamines (Berry et al., 1942; Bronk et al., 1939). Local vasoconstriction in blood vessels has been observed when the hypothalamus is stimulated (Eliasson et al., 1952, 1954). These responses to stimulation are mediated by the brain-stem pressor mechanisms (Alexander, 1946; Lindgren, 1955; McQueen et al., 1954; Wang and Ranson, 1939).

When the hypothalamus is stimulated, adrenergic (vasoconstrictor) discharge is distributed to the entire vascular bed with the exception of skeletal muscle, in which vasodilatation occurs (Eichna and McQuarrie, 1960; Eliasson et al., 1952, 1954; Lindgren, 1955; Lindgren and Uvnäs, 1954; Uvnäs, 1960). The same effects on the vascular bed occur when vasoconstrictor fibers are activated by cerebral cortical stimulation (Löfving, 1961).

Hypothalamic stimulation also elicits a behavioral response called the "defense" reaction, first described by Hess (1949) in the cat. During this reaction sympathetically mediated vasodilation occurs in muscle, accompanied by an increased heart rate, vasoconstriction in vascular beds other than muscle, and the increased secretion of catecholamines (Abrahams et al., 1960) and ACTH (Folkow et al., 1965). When the defense reaction is elicited, the cat growls, hisses, runs, and its pupils are dilated and its fur stands up (Hess, 1949; Hunsperger, 1956). The reaction is brought about by stimulation of the hypothalamus near the entrance of the fornix, the dorsomedial amygdala, and the striae terminalis (Fernandez de Molina and Hunsperger, 1959, 1962). The cerebral cortex in turn attenuates the violence of the defense reaction produced by stimulation of the hypothalamic sites. Repetitive stimulation of the same site permanently increases blood pressure levels in some animals. Folkow and Rubinstein (1966) produced sustained hypertension in rats by mild and intermittent daily stimulation, for several months, of the perifornical area of the hypothalamus. The implications of this study are manifold. Folkow (1971) has pointed out that activation of this area of the brain leads to dilatation of the blood vessels in muscle and constriction of the renal circulation to produce the release of renin and angiotensin, which, in turn, may act directly on the brain stem to raise the blood pressure.

The Regulation of Blood Pressure and Peripheral Resistance by the Central Nervous System

Central to our current notions about the regulation of blood pressure by the brain is that changes in vasomotor tone are brought about by variations in vasoconstrictor activity: decreased vasoconstrictor discharge leads to vasodilation and a fall in blood pressure, increased discharge to vasoconstriction and an increase in the blood pressure (Folkow and Uvnäs, 1950; Lindgren and Uvnäs, 1954). Vasoconstrictor tone is partly controlled by afferent impulses passing from the carotid sinus baroreceptors and aortic arch

83

mechanoreceptors that respond to increased in arterial pCO_2. Stimulation of the baroreceptors leads to vasoconstriction (Heymans and Neil, 1958). The mechanoreceptors respond to their pulsatile distension (Ead et al., 1952) and to the rate with which changes in arterial pressure occur (Peterson, 1961). From the carotid mechanoreceptors, afferent impulses pass via the sinus nerve to the medullary vasomotor centers. The mechanoreceptors usually discharge in rhythmic bursts, beginning with the start of systole and ending as the pulse wave passes (Douglas et al., 1956; Douglas and Ritchie, 1956; Landgren, 1952). When the arterial pressure is high, neural discharge is sustained not phasic (Bronk and Stella, 1932). Adaptation to the high pressures occurs eventually so that neural discharge diminishes in rate. As a result of this adaptation the high blood pressure is not reflexly reduced.

Tonic neuronal activity in the sinus nerve is always present; cutting the sinus nerve immediately raises the blood pressure. Therefore, afferent tonic activity in the sinus nerve reflexly inhibits vasoconstrictor tone and continually prevents the blood pressure from rising.

Other afferent impulses also arise from receptors in the atrial walls of the heart and ventricles and from the walls of the great veins. All afferent neuronal activity from the various receptors in the heart and great vessels pass to the vasomotor centers in the medulla oblongata. The vasomotor centers also receive neuronal input from other parts of the body through sympathetic afferent fibers that first enter the spinal cord. The fibers travel up an ipsilateral pathway in the fasciculus gracilis and a bilateral one in the anterolateral portion of the cord. These pathways reach the posterior hypothalamus, the thalamus, and the cerebral cortex and act as the afferent arm of circuits that eventually feed back into the vasomotor center (Amassian, 1951; Downman, 1955). Afferent baroreceptor and mechanoreceptor impulses first pass to the nucleus of the tractus solitarius (NTS) in the medulla. From this nucleus, inhibitory neurons pass to the pressor vasomotor center, and excitatory neurons pass to the depressor center. Inhibitory catecholaminergic neurons also enter the depressor center. These catecholaminergic neurons probably originate from the higher parts of the brain stem and hypothalamus. Other catecholaminergic neurons from higher centers pass to the NTS (Fuxe, 1965) and to the pressor center. Their exact function is not known. Destruction of the NTS releases the pressor center from inhibition, and high blood pressure levels occur (Doba and Reis, 1973, 1974). The pressor center lies in the lateral reticular formation of the rostral two-thirds of the medulla oblongata. The depressor center lies medially and caudally in the reticular formation of the medulla (Alexander, 1946; Korner, 1971; Ranson and Billingsley, 1916). Tonic inhibitory impulses to spinal vasomotor mechanisms emanate from the depressor zone (Wang and Ranson, 1939). These inhibitory neurons may be serotonergic (Neumayr et al., 1974). The neurons of both centers are constantly active (Alexander, 1946). Tonic excitatory influences mediated by noradrenergic neurons from the pressor area impinge on spinal vasomotor neurons (Chalmers and Wurtman, 1971). The synaptic events at spinal vasomotor neurons causing increased or decreased discharge are not known (Humphrey, 1967).

The intensity of the discharge in preganglionic vasoconstrictor neurons is the resultant of the excitatory and inhibitory tonic impulses that flow from the brain stem (Alexander, 1945). The frequency of tonic discharge in vasoconstrictor nerves is low (Bronk et al., 1936; Celander and Folkow, 1953; Folkow, 1952); the discharge occurs in rhythmic

84

bursts, in concert with the pulse beat and the respiratory rhythm (Dontas, 1955). The fall in arterial blood pressure on activation of the baroreceptor reflex causes a decrease in spinal sympathetic neuronal discharge, diminished activity in noradrenergic postganglionic nerves, vasodilation in muscle, the splanchnic bed, and the skin (von Euler, 1956; Folkow et al, 1950; Uvnäs, 1960).

Acute and chronic elevations in arterial pressure—neurogenic hypertension—results from denervation of the baroreceptors and mechanoreceptors (Hering, 1923; Koch, 1931). In experimental neurogenic hypertension blood pressure levels fluctuate wildly and tachycardia occurs. Destruction of central noradrenergic and dopaminergic neurons by 6-hydroxydopamine both prevents the development and "cures" established neurogenic hypertension (Chalmers and Wurtman, 1971). Destruction of central serotonergic neurons also prevents neurogenic hypertension (Wing and Chalmers, 1974).

Denervating the baroreceptors and producing neurogenic hypertension is an instructive experiment that does not necessarily prove that the baroreceptors play a role in the pathogenesis of essential hypertension. In human hypertension the carotid sinus (baroreceptor) reflex remains active and functioning, but the baroreceptors gradually adapt to high blood pressure levels and no longer act maximally to reduce them. The adaptation occurs in dogs within one to two days after a renal artery is clamped to produce high blood pressure (McCubbin, 1958), and it is characterized by an increase both in the threshold and a decrease in the range of response to stimulation. The sinus nerve shows a decrease in hypertensive animals (McCubbin et al., 1956). The adaptation to high blood pressure levels may be due to the direct effect of the high systemic arterial pressures rather than to some chemical substance that is liberated (Kezdi, 1962). The adaptation of the baroreceptors to an elevated mean blood pressure would act to sustain it; the decrease in afferent discharge would lead to a decreased inhibition of vasomotor tone and, therefore, to vasoconstriction. Therapeutic measures have been devised to counteract baroreceptor adaptation in human hypertension. Electrical stimulation of the sinus nerve (to restore neural activity after adaptation) lowers blood pressure in hypertensive patients (Bilgutay and Lillehei, 1965; Schwartz and Griffith, 1967).

In addition to lowering the blood pressure, stimulating the baroreceptors by stretching has effects on the brain. Bonvallet et al. (1956) distended the carotid sinus while keeping the blood pressure at a constant level. They produced synchronization of the electroencephalogram (EEG). They believe that an increase in afferent activity occludes the tonic, corticopetal, desynchronizing influences of the midbrain reticular-activating formation. Therefore, it is possible that when baroreceptor adaptation occurs in human hypertension, cortical desynchronization and behavioral arousal might be produced.

Elevated blood pressure levels affect the brain directly, in addition to those effects mediated by mechanoreceptors. Thus, Baust et al. (1963) have reported that raising the blood pressure directly causes desynchronization of the EEG in the *encephale isolé* cat, by virtue of its effect on the mesencephalic reticular formation. The mechanical effect of a rise in blood pressure may cause the firing rate of single posterior hypothalamic and mesencephalic reticular neurons to increase (Baust and Katz, 1961; Baust et al., 1962). This mechanical stimulus to the brain may also cause the release of humoral substances, such as vasopressin.

This brief review of the brain mechanisms involved in cardiovascular regulation suggests that medullary and spinal vasomotor neurons are reflexly controlled by afferent input from mechanoreceptors, but are also powerfully influenced by sensory inputs, by motor mechanisms, and by numerous circuits from diverse areas of the brain. In addition to the classical vasomotor mechanisms, a separate sympathetic vasodilator system has been described (Eliasson et al., 1952, 1954; Lindgren, 1955; Löfving, 1961; Uvnäs, 1960). This second system may be responsible for the integrated motor and circulatory changes seen with exercise and difficult intellectual tasks. Activation of this system produces phasic constriction of the splanchnic bed and increases in blood pressure. It is not yet known whether such changes are related to the onset of hypertension. Perhaps the only certainty is that the central nervous system is involved in sustaining high levels of blood pressure due to adaptation of the baroreceptors, and that a lowering of blood pressure occurs when the sinus nerve is stimulated electrically.

The increased appetite for salt in patients with hypertension, the confirmed evidence of the action of angiotensin II on the brain stem, and the regulation of the adrenal cortex and medulla by the hypothalmic-pituitary axis all point to the participation of the central nervous system in some phase of essential hypertension.

SUMMARY AND CONCLUSIONS

Anyone attempting to assess the current status of this field must hesitate in making any definitive statement about the predisposition to, initiation of, and sustaining factors in high blood pressure. Such a hesitation is occasioned by the realization that many of the most hallowed ideas about essential hypertension have undergone drastic revision in the past 20 years. It was once believed that cardiac output was normal in patients with essential hypertension who were not in cardiac failure. This belief has been shattered by the observation of an enhanced cardiac output in some patients with an early, "labile" form of the illness, who have borderline elevations of blood pressure.

The implication of this finding is that the initial phase of the disease is different in different patients. Presumably, different physiological mechanisms underlie different forms of the initial phase of the disease. In borderline, labile hypertension, the increased cardiac output seems to be due to increased β-adrenergic sympathetic stimulation of the heart. In other forms of early high blood pressure, plasma renin levels may be elevated. Still other hypertensive patients have a low plasma renin activity. Essential hypertension can also occur in association with normal plasma renin activity. But the interesting aspect of the relationship of plasma renin activity to essential hypertension is not the level of this enzyme's activity, but the fact that in many patients there are a variety of disturbances in the regulation of aldosterone by renin and its product, angiotensin II.

Shapiro (1973) has pointed out that with the exception of reninomas, pheo-chromocytomas, and aldosterinomas, no single physiological disturbance will fully account for the elevated blood pressure of essential hypertension in all its forms. The conclusion that does emerge at the present time is that essential hypertension comes about by a variety of disturbances in the relationship between the various systems involved in the regulation of blood pressure. Essential hypertension is a heterogeneous condition brought about by various mechanisms. No single cause, or single change in the level of a hormone or enzyme, will explain the etiology, pathogenesis, or pathophysiology of all forms of essential hypertension. The disturbances in the mechanisms of blood pressure regulation are different at different stages of the disease, and in different stages in its subgroups. These general conclusions are supported by work on animals. High blood pressure can be produced by many different experimental manipulations—from altering the early social experiences of the animal to constricting one renal artery. Not all strains of one species of animals respond with high blood pressure to the same experimental manipulation. The same experimental procedure also produces high blood pressure in one animal genus and not another. And when members of different animal genera are subjected to the same procedure the mechanisms that produce high blood pressure differ.

In animals high blood pressure can be produced by varying their early and later social experiences. These experiences also affect the neurochemistry of the brain and the later behavior of these animals. The brain mediates the effects of social experiences. It also mediates the effect of desoxycorticosterone acetate and salt treatment of rats, the hypertensive effects of carotid sinus denervation, and the initiation of high blood pressure in the spontaneously hypertensive rat. The brain, through its regulation of vasomotor tone participates in the initiation of these various forms of high blood pressure in different ways. Once high blood pressure levels are instituted, other mechanisms in the body may sustain them.

These conclusions are relevant to the discussion of psychological factors in essential hypertension. In a general way, animal experiments support the notion that social and psychological factors in human beings may play an etiological and pathogenetic role in essential hypertension. These experiments underline the importance of prior experience and of social conflict in producing high blood pressure, renal disease, and changes in brain and adrenal neurotransmitter substances and their biosynthetic enzymes. They support the idea that these physiological changes are the consequences of changes in social conditions and behavior. A note of caution must be introduced at this point. Social and psychological factors may play a role in some but not all subgroups of the disease. Alternatively, these factors may play more of a role in some but not all forms of the disease, or at some stage of the disease and not at other stages. For example, the inception of the malignant phase of essential hypertension has been correlated with changes in the personal life of hypertensive patients or in the doctor-patient relationship.

Psychosocial factors do not by themselves "cause" essential hypertension. Genetic factors also predispose to the disease. Even the high blood pressure of renovascular disease is usually associated with a family history of high blood pressure (Shapiro, 1973; Shapiro et al., 1969). The exact nature of these family factors is unknown. They may or may not be genetic.

The social environment seems to play a major role in preventing or facilitating the development of high blood pressure in genetically predisposed human beings. Social injustice, dislocation and disruption, physical danger, violence, marital discord, separation, and poverty promote high blood pressure, fear, and rage. Social stability is conducive to blood pressure levels that remain even throughout a person's life.

Some patients with high blood pressure levels are particularly sensitive and alert to danger, violence, lack of tact, scorn, and malevolence in others. Some patients may be able to cope with tactlessness or danger by not being aware of or disregarding them. When this method of coping no longer works, the patients become afraid and angry.

Many hypertensives do seem to be vigilant to danger, unwilling to engage in close personal interaction, and particularly sensitive to potentially hostile interactions with others. They may superficially appear to be submissive, inhibited in expressing aggressive or hostile thoughts, or in engaging in hostile deeds. In any case, no one personality type is predisposed to essential hypertension. Some hypertensive patients are submissive, and some are provocative, challenging, and combative.

Anger is frequently present in patients with high blood pressure levels. But we cannot assume that anger "causes" high blood pressure. Anger might result from the high blood pressure or the physiological changes that accompany it. Future experiments could test these alternative views. The hypothesis that conflicts about anger antecede the development of essential hypertension should also be tested before the high blood pressure levels develop or in patients with borderline, labile hypertension. But predictive studies cannot be carried out without knowing the nature of the risk factors of this disease. In patients with labile hypertension, studies to determine the psychological, social, and dietary factors in producing an increase in β-adrenergic sympathetic stimulus to the heart should be carried out. The everyday events that produce increases in blood pressure, cardiac output, and heart rate in these patients should be recorded. Everyday events and the psychological responses to them do correspond to profound blood pressure changes in patients with established hypertension. Even banal events in the lives of these patients can correspond to excessive blood pressure changes.

We cannot as yet be certain that in man social and psychological factors are the antecedents, and not the consequences, of the altered physiological changes in essential hypertension. Experiments in animals that later develop high blood pressure point up the important role of prior experience, but in some animals, stressful experiences do not initiate high blood pressure, but determine its level. Two conclusions can be drawn from these experiments.

First, early experiences of the future hypertensive patient may be etiologically relevant. Much more needs to be known about the childhood experiences and the families of persons who later develop essential hypertension. For example, the reasons for the family aggregation of essential hypertension are unknown. We might ask whether parents of the future patient do not also display the same perceptual and interpersonal styles and sensitivities that have been described in hypertensive patients themselves. If so, how do such parents affect their children?

Second, psychological factors are known to play a role in altering the course of the disease. Separation may antecede the malignant phase. Other factors such as excessive renin activity, a renal infection, and excessive salt and water intake in the presence of long-standing changes in the kidney may also antecede the accelerated, malignant phase. Therefore, the course of the disease may be altered not by any particular factor but by one of many, or by a combination of factors.

This chapter has attempted to bring to the attention of behavioral scientists the complex factors that are involved in elevating blood pressure levels. Essential hypertension seems to be a multifactorial and heterogeneous disease. Bias in, or disturbance of any of the mechanisms regulating blood pressure levels may set off a chain of events that end in high blood pressure. The disturbance may begin with changes in cardiac output, peripheral resistance, the kidney adrenal cortex or medulla, or the brain. Once the disturbance starts, the other mechanisms regulating blood pressure are altered.

It would have been desirable, if possible, to have made a definitive statement about the role of psychological factors in essential hypertension: however, no such statement can be made. Psychological factors clearly do not by themselves "cause" the syndrome. These factors interact with the other predispositions to high blood pressure. In some persons, the social factors and the psychological responses they provoke may interact with a biased system, such as an altered regulation of aldosterone by renin and angiotensin. In other persons these psychosocial factors may increase β-adrenergic discharge to the heart, cardiac output, and, finally, the peripheral resistance, to produce high blood pressure.

In still other patients, social conditions, separation, anxiety, and anger may potentiate and aggravate an already increased blood pressure level and vascular hyperreactivity. The inferences can be drawn from the accumulated knowledge about essential hypertension that it is a disease that can be brought about by many different mechanisms, and that social and psychological factors may play a different etiological, pathogenetic, and sustaining role in its different forms.

REFERENCES

Abrahams, V. C., and Pickford, M. 1956. Observations on a central antagonism between adrenaline and acetylcholine. *J. Physiol.* (Lond.) 131:712.

———, Hilton, S. M., and Zbrozyna, A. 1960. Active muscle vasodilation produced by stimulation of the brain stem: Its significance in the defence reaction. *J. Physiol.* (Lond.) 154:491.

Abramson, D. I. 1944. *Vascular responses in the extremities of man in health and disease.* Chicago: University of Chicago Press.

——— and Ferris, E. B., Jr. 1940. Responses of blood vessels in the resting hand and forearm to various stimuli. *Am. Heart J.* 19:541.

Aceto, M. D. G., Kinnard, W. J., and Buckley, J. P. 1963. Effect of compounds on blood pressure and behavioural response of rats chronically subjected to an avoidance escape situation. *Arch. Int. Pharmacodyn. Ther.* 144:214.

Acheson, R. M., and Fowler, G. B. 1967. On the inheritance of stature and blood pressure. *J. Chronic Dis.* 20:731.

Adams, D. B., Baccelli, G., Mancia, G., and Zanchetti, A. 1968. Cardiovascular changes during preparation for fighting behavior in the cat. *Nature* 220:1239.

Aleksandrow, D. 1967. Studies on the epidemiology of hypertension in Poland. In *The Epidemiology of Hypertension*, edited by J. Stamler, R. Stamler, and T. N. Pullman. New York: Grune & Stratton.

Alexander, F. 1939. Psychoanalytic study of a case of essential hypertension. *Psychosom. Med.* 1:139.

——— 1950. *Psychosomatic Medicine.* New York: Norton.

———, French, T. M., and Pollock, G. H. 1968. *Psychosomatic Specificity.* Chicago: University of Chicago Press.

Alexander, R. S. 1945. The effects of blood flow and anoxia on spinal cardiovascular centers. *Am. J. Physiol.* 143:698.

——— 1946. Tonic and reflex functions of medullary sympathetic cardiovascular centers. *J. Neurophysiol.* 9:205.

Amassian, V. E. 1951. Fiber groups and spinal pathways of cortically represented visceral afferents. *J. Neurophysiol.* 14:445.

Ames, R. P.; Borkowski, A. W., Sicinski, A. M., and Laragh, J. H. 1965. Prolonged infusions of angiotensin II and norepinephrine and blood pressure, electrolyte balance, and aldosterone and cortisol secretion in normal man and in cirrhosis with ascites. *J. Clin. Invest.* 44:1171.

Anand, B. K., and Dua, S. 1956a. Circulatory and respiratory changes induced by electrical stimulation of limbic system (visceral brain). *J. Neurophysiol.* 19:393.

———— and ———— 1956b. Electrical stimulation of the limbic system of brain (visceral brain) in the waking animals. *Indian J. Med. Res.* 44:107.

Andén, N. E., Carrodi, H., Dahlström, A., Fuxe, K., and Hökfelt, J. 1966. Effects of tyrosine hydroxylase inhibition on the amine levels of central monamine levels. *Life Sci.* 5:561.

Anderson, D. E., and Brady, J. V. 1971. Pre-avoidance blood pressure elevations accompanied by heart rate decreases in the dog. *Science* 172:595.

———— and ———— 1973. Prolonged pre-avoidance effects upon blood pressure and heart rate in the dog. *Psychosom. Med.* 35:4.

Andersson, B., and McCann, S. M. 1955. A further study of polydipsia evoked by hypothalamic stimulation in the goat. *Acta Physiol. Scand.* 33:333.

Andreev, S. V., Vadkovskaia, I. D., and Glebova, M. S. 1952. Effect of renin preparations on the blood pressure. *Tr. Akad. Med. Nauk. Gipertonicheskaia Bolezn.* 2:56.

Armstrong, J. G. 1959. Hypotensive action of progesterone in experimental and human hypertension. *Proc. Soc. Exp. Biol. Med.* 102:452.

Arnold, P., and Rosenheim, M. I. 1949. Effect of pentamethonium iodide on normal and hypertensive persons. *Lancet* 257:321.

Asafov, B. D. 1958. *The Orienting Reflex and Exploratory Behavior.* Moscow: Akad. Ped. Nauk RSFSR.

August, J. T., Nelson, D. H., and Thorn, G. W. 1958. Response of normal subjects to large amounts of aldosterone. *J. Clin. Invest.* 37:1549.

Ax, A. F. 1953. The physiological differentiation between fear and anger in humans. *Psychosom. Med.* 15:433.

Ayers, C. B., Harris, R. H., Jr., and Lefer, L. G. 1969. Control of renin release in experimental hypertension. *Circ. Res.* 34 (Suppl. I): I–103.

Ayitey-Smith, E., and Varma, D. R. 1970. Assessment of the role of the sympathetic nervous system in experimental hypertension using normal and immunosympathectomised rats. *Br. J. Pharmacol.* 40:175.

Ayman, D. 1930. An evaluation of therapeutic results in essential hypertension. *J.A.M.A.* 95:246.

———— 1933. The personality type of patients with arteriolar essential hypertension. *Am. J. Med. Sci.* 186:213.

———— 1934. Heredity in arteriolar (essential) hypertension: a clinical study of the blood pressure of 1,524 members of 277 families. *Arch. Intern. Med.* 53:792.

———— and Pratt, J. H. 1931. Nature of the symptoms associated with essential hypertension. *Arch. Intern. Med.* 47:675.

Baer, L., Sommers, S. C., Krakoff, L. R., Newton, M. A., and Laragh, J. H. 1970. Pseudo-primary aldosteronism: an entity distinct from true primary aldosteronism. *Circ. Res.* 26–27 (Suppl. I):203.

Baldwin, D. S., Biggs, A. W., Goldring, W., Hulet, W. M., and Chasis, H. 1958. Exaggerated natriuresis in essential hypertension. *Am. J. Med.* 24:893.

Ball, C. O. T., and Meneely, G. R. 1957. Observations on dietary sodium chloride. *J. Am. Diet. Assoc.* 33:366.

Barach, J. H. 1928. The constitutional factors in hypertensive disease. *J.A.M.A.* 91:1511.

Barbour, B. H., Slater, J. D. H., Casper, A. G. I., and Bartter, F. C. 1965. On the role of the central nervous system in control of aldosterone secretion. *Life Sci.* 4:1161.

Barcroft, H., Brod, J., Hejl, Z., Hirsjarvi, E. A., and Kitchin, A. H. 1960. The mechanism of the vasodilatation in the forearm muscle during stress (mental arithmetic). *Clin. Sci.* 19:577.

90

Bartter, F. C., Mills, I. H., Biglieri, E. G., and Delia, C. 1959. Studies on the control and physiologic action of aldosterone. *Recent Prog. Horm. Res.* 15:311.

——, ——, and Gann, D. S. 1960. Increase in aldosterone secretion by carotid artery constriction in the dog and its prevention by thyrocarotid arterial function denervation. *J. Clin. Invest.* 39:1330.

Bassett, D. R., Rosenblatt, G., Moellerung, R. D., and Hartwell, A. S. 1966. Cardiovascular disease, diabetes mellitus and anthropometric evaluation of Polynesian males on the Island of Niihau—1963. *Circulation* 34:1088.

Baust, W., and Katz, P. 1961. Untersuchung zur Tonisierung einzelner Neurone im hinteren Hypothalamus. *Pflügers Arch.* 272:575.

——, Niemczyk, H., Schaeffer, H., and Vieth, J. 1962. On a pressor sensitive area in the posterior hypothalamus of cats. *Pflügers Arch.* 274:374.

——, ——, and Vieth, J. 1963. The action of blood pressure on the ascending reticular activating system with special reference to adrenaline-induced EEG arousal. *Electroencephogr. Clin. Neurophysiol.* 15:63.

Bays, R. P., and Scrimshaw, N. S. 1953. Facts and fallacies regarding the blood pressure of different regional and racial groups. *Circulation* 8:655.

Beavers, W. R., and Blackmore, W. P. 1958. Effect of chlorothiazide on vascular reactivity. *Proc. Soc. Exp. Biol. Med.* 98:133.

Bechgaard, P. 1967. The natural history of benign hypertension: one thousand hypertensive patients followed from 26 to 32 years. In *The Epidemiology of Essential Hypertension*, edited by J. Stamler, R. Stamler, and T. N. Pullman. New York: Grune & Stratton.

Beier, D. C. 1940. Conditioned cardiovascular responses and suggestions for treatment of cardiac neuroses. *J. Exp. Psychol.* 26:311.

Bello, C. T., Sevy, R. W., Harakal, C., and Hillyer, P. N. 1967. Relationship between clinical severity of disease and hemodynamic patterns in essential hypertension. *Am. J. Med. Sci.* 253:194.

Benedict, R. 1956. Onset and early course of essential hypertension. *J. Chron. Dis.* 4:221.

Benson, H., Herd, J. A., Morse, W. H., and Kelleher, R. T. 1969. Behavioral induction of arterial hypertension and its reversal. *Am. J. Physiol.* 217:30.

——, ——, ——, and —— 1970. Behaviorally induced hypertension in the squirrel monkey. *Circ. Res.* 26–27 (Suppl. I):I–21.

——, Shapiro, D., Tursky, B., and Schwartz, G. E. 1971. Decreased systolic blood pressure through operant conditioning techniques in patients with essential hypertension. *Science* 173:740.

Benson, W. R., and Sealy, W. C. 1956. Arterial necrosis following resection of coarctation of the aorta. *Lab. Invest.* 5:359.

Berkson, D. M., Stamler, J., Lindberg, H. A., Miller, W., Mathias, H., Lasky, H., and Hall, Y. 1960. Socioeconomic correlates of atherosclerotic and hypertensive heart disease. *Ann. N.Y. Acad. Sci.* 84:835.

Berry, C., McKinley, W., and Hodes, R. 1942. Reversals of blood pressure responses caused by changes in frequency of brain stem stimulation. *Am. J. Physiol.* 135:338.

Bianchi, G., Tenconi, L. T., and Lucca, R. 1970. Effect in the conscious dog of constriction of the renal artery to a sole remaining kidney on haemodynamics, sodium balance, body fluid volumes, plasma renin concentration and pressor responsiveness to angiotensin. *Clin. Sci. Mol. Med.* 38:741.

Biglieri, E. G., Slaton, P. E., Jr., Kronefield, S. J., and Deck, J. B. 1967. Primary aldosteronism with unusual secretory pattern. *J. Clin. Endocrinol. Metab.* 27:715.

Bilgutay, A. M., and Lillehei, C. W. 1965. Treatment of hypertension with an implantable electronic device. *J.A.M.A.* 191:649.

Bing, J., and Poulsen, K. 1970. Effect of anti-angiotensin II on blood pressure and sensitivity to angiotensin and renin. *Acta Path. Microbiol. Scand.* [A] 78:6.

——— and Vinthen-Paulsen, N. 1952. Effects of severe anoxia on the kidneys of normal and dehydrated mice. *Acta Physiol. Scand.* 27:337.

Binger, C. A., Ackerman, N. W., Cohn, A. E., Schroeder, H. A., and Steele, J. M. 1945. *Personality in Arterial Hypertension.* New York: Brunner.

Biron, P., Koiw, E., Nowaczynski, W., Brouillet, J., and Genest, J. 1961. The effects of intravenous infusions of valine-5 angiotensin II and other pressor agents on urinary electrolytes and corticosteroids, including aldosterone. *J. Clin. Invest.* 40:338.

Blair, D. A., Glover, W. E., Greenfield, A. D. M., and Roddie, I. C. 1959. Excitation of cholinergic vasodilator nerves to human skeletal muscles during emotional states. *J. Physiol.* (Lond.) 148:633.

Blair-West, J. R., Coghlan, J. P., Denton, D. A., Orchard, E., Scoggins, B. A., and Wright, R. D. 1968a. Renin-angiotensin-aldosterone system and sodium balance in experimental renal hypertension. *Endocrinology* 83:119.

———, ———, ———, Funder, J. W., Scoggins, B. A., and Wright, R. D. 1968b. Effects of adrenal steroid withdrawal on chronic renovascular hypertension in adrenalectomized sheep. *Circ. Res.* 23:803.

Blanchard, E. B., and Young, L. D. 1973. Self-control of cardiac functioning: A promise as yet unfulfilled. *Psychol. Bull.* 79:145.

Bliss, E. L., and Zwanziger, J. 1966. Brain amines and emotional stress. *J. Psychiat. Res.* 4:189.

Bøe, J., Humerfelt, S., and Wedervang, F. 1957. Blood pressure in a population. *Acta Med. Scand.* 157 (Suppl. 321):1.

Bock, K. D., and Krecke, H. J. 1958. Die Wirkung von syntetischem Hypertensin II auf die PAH—und Inulin—clearance, die renale Hemodynamik und die Diurese beim Menschen. *Klin. Wschr.* 36:69.

Bonvallet, M., Hugelin, A., and Dell, P. 1956. The interior environment and automatic activities of the reticular cells of the mesencephalon. *J. Physiol.* (Paris) 48:403.

Booth, D. A. 1968. Mechanism of action of norepinephrine in eliciting an eating response on injection into the rat hypothalamus. *J. Pharmacol. Exp. Ther.* 160:336.

Boucher, R., Asselin, J., and Genest, J. 1974. A new enzyme leading to the direct formation of angiotensin II. *Circ. Res.* 34 (Suppl. I):I–203.

Bourgault, P. C., Karczmar, A. G., and Scudder, C. L. 1963. Contrasting behavioral, pharmacological, neurophysiological, and biochemical profiles of C57BL/6 and SC-I strains of mice. *Life Sci.* 8:533.

Boyd, J. E., and Mulrow, P. J. 1972. Intracellular potassium: the regulator of aldosterone production. *J. Clin. Invest.* 51:13a.

Braun-Menendez, E., and von Euler, U. S. 1947. Hypertension after bilateral nephrectomy in the rat. *Nature* 160:905.

Brod, J. 1960. Essential hypertension—hemodynamic observations with bearing on its pathogenesis. *Lancet* ii:773.

——— 1970. Hemodynamics and emotional stress. *Bibl. Psychiatr.* 144:13.

———, Fenčl, V., Hejl, Z., and Jirka, J. 1959. Circulatory changes underlying blood pressure elevation during acute emotional stress (mental arithmetic) in normotensive and hypertensive subjects. *Clin. Sci.* 18:269.

———, ———, ———, ———, and Ulrych, M. 1962. General and regional hemodynamic pattern underlying essential hypertension. *Clin. Sci.* 23:339.

Brodie, B. B., and Costa, E. 1961. Role of norepinephrine in peripheral ganglia on blood pressure.

In *Hypertension—Recent Advances: The Second Hahnemann Symposium on Hypertensive Disease,* edited by A. N. Brest and J. H. Moyer. Philadelphia: Lea & Febiger.

Bronk, D. W., and Stella, G. 1932. Afferent impulses in the carotid sinus nerve. *J. Cell Physiol.* 1:113.

———, Pitts, R. F., and Larrabee, M. G. 1939. Role of hypothalamus in cardiovascular regulation. *Res. Publ. Assoc. Nerv. Ment. Dis.* 20:323.

Bronson, F. H. 1967. Effects of social stimulation on adrenal and reproductive physiology of rodents. In *Husbandry of Laboratory Animals,* edited by M. L. Conalty. New York: Academic.

Brooks, C. McC., Ushiyama, J., and Lange, G. 1962. Reactions of neurons in or near the supraoptic nuclei. *Am. J. Physiol.* 202:487.

Brower, D. 1947a. The relation between certain Rorschach factors and cardiovascular activity before and after visuo-motor conflict. *J. Gen. Psychol.* 37:93.

——— 1947b. The relations between Minnesota Multiphasic Personality Inventory scores and cardiovascular measures before and after experimentally induced visuo-motor conflict. *J. Soc. Psychol.* 26:55.

Brown, T. C., Davis, J. O., Olichney, M. J., and Johnston, C. I. 1966. Relation of plasma renin to sodium balance and arterial pressure in experimental renal hypertension. *Circ. Res.* 18:475.

Bruce, J. M., Jr., and Thomas, C. B. 1953. A method of rating certain personality factors as determined by the Rorschach test for use in a study of the precursors of hypertension and coronary artery disease. *Psychiatr. Q.* 27(Suppl.):207.

Brunner, H. R., Baer, L., Sealey, J. E., Ledingham, J. G. G., and Laragh, J. H. 1970. The influence of potassium administration and of potassium deprivation on plasma renin in normal and hypertensive subjects. *J. Clin, Invest.* 49:2128.

———, Kirshman, J. D., Sealey, J. E., and Laragh, J. H. 1971. Hypertension of renal origin. Evidence for two different mechanisms. *Science* 174:1344.

———, Laragh, J. H., Baer, L., Newton, M. A., Goodwin, F. T., Krakoff, L. R., Bard, R. H., and Buhler, F. R. 1972. Essential hypertension: renin and aldosterone, heart attack and stroke. *N. Engl. J. Med.* 286:441.

Bunag, R. D., Page, I. H., and McCubbin, J. W. 1966. Neural stimulation of release of renin. *Circ. Res.* 19:851.

Buss, A. H. 1961. *The Psychology of Aggression.* New York: Wiley.

Bykov, K. M. 1947. *The Cerebral Cortex and the Internal Organs.* Moscow: Medgiz.

Byrom, F. B., and Dodson, L. F. 1949. Mechanism of the vicious cycle in chronic hypertension. *Clin. Sci.* 8:1.

Cannon, P. J., Ames, R. P., and Laragh, J. H. 1966. Relation between potassium balance and aldosterone secretion in normal subjects and in patients with hypertensive or renal tubular disease. *J. Clin. Invest.* 45:865.

Cannon, W. B. 1929. *Bodily Changes in Pain, Hunger, Fear and Rage.* New York: Appleton-Century-Crofts.

Carpenter, C. C. J., Davis, J. O., and Ayers, C. R. 1961a, Concerning the role of arterial baroreceptors in the control of aldosterone secretion. *J. Clin. Invest.* 40:1160.

———, ———, and ——— 1961b. Relation of renin, angiotensin II, and experimental renal hypertension to aldosterone secretion. *J. Clin. Invest.* 40:2026.

Carretero, O. A., Kuk, P., Bujak, B., and Houle, J. 1971. Effect of antibodies against angiotensin II on the blood pressure of rats with severe experimental hypertension. *Fed. Proc.* 30:432.

Catt, K. J., Kimmet, P. Z., Cain, M. D., Cran, E., Best, J. B., and Coghlan, J. P. 1971. Angiotensin II blood levels in human hypertension. *Lancet* i:459.

Cattell, R. B., and Scheier, I. H. 1959. Extension of meaning of objective test personality factors:

Especially into anxiety, neuroticism, questionnaire, and physical factors. *J. Gen. Psychol.* 61:287.

Celander, O. 1954. The range of control exercised by the sympathico-adrenal system: a quantive study on blood vessels and other smooth muscle effectors in the cat. *Acta Physiol. Scand.* (Suppl. 32):116:1.

———— and Folkow, B. 1953. A comparison of the sympathetic vasomotor fibre control of the vessels within the skin and the muscles. *Acta Physiol. Scand.* 29:241.

Chalmers, J. P. 1975. Brain amines and models of experimental hypertension. *Circ. Res.* 36:469.

Chalmers, J. P., and Wurtman, R. J. 1971. Participation of central noradrenergic neurons in arterial baroreceptor reflexes in the rabbit. *Circ. Res.* 28:480.

Chambers, W. W., and Reiser, M. F. 1953. Emotional stress in the precipitation of congestive heart failure. *Psychosom. Med.* 15:38.

Charvat, J., Dell, P., and Folkow, B. 1964. Mental factors and cardiovascular diseases. *Cardiologia* 44:124.

Chobanian, A. V., Burrows, B. A., and Hollander, W. 1961. Body fluid and electrolyte composition in arterial hypertension. II. Studies in mineralocorticoid hypertension. *J. Clin. Invest.* 40:416.

Christenson, W. N., and Hinkle, L. E. 1961. Differences in illness and prognostic signs in two groups of young men. *J.A.M.A.* 177:247.

Christian, J. J., Lloyd, J. A., and Davis, D. 1965. The role of endocrines in the self-regulation of mammalian populations. *Recent Prog. Horm. Res.* 22:501.

Christiansen, J., Hagerup, L., and Nielsen, B. 1964. Hypokalemia and hypertension. *Acta Med. Scand.* 176:665.

Christlieb, A. R., Biber, T. U. L., and Hickler, R. B. 1969. Studies on the role of angiotensin in experimental renovascular hypertension: an immunologic approach. *J. Clin. Invest.* 48:1506.

Christy, N. P., and Laragh, J. H. 1961. Pathogenesis of hypokalemic alkalosis in Cushing's syndrome. *N. Engl. J. Med.* 265:1083.

Cohen, S. I., and Silverman, A. J. 1959. Psychophysiological investigations of vascular response variability. *J. Psychosom. Res.* 3:185.

————, ————, Zuidema, G., and Lazar, C. 1957. Psychotherapeutic alteration of a physiologic stress response. *J. Nerv. Ment. Dis.* 125:112.

Coleman, T. G., and Guyton, A. C. 1969. Hypertension caused by salt loading in the dog. III. Onset transients of cardiac output and other variables. *Circ. Res.* 25:153.

Comstock, G. W. 1957. An epidemiologic study of blood pressure levels in a biracial community in the Southern United States. *Am. J. Hyg.* 65:271.

Conn, J. W. 1955. Part II. Primary aldosteronism, a new clinical syndrome. *J. Lab. Clin. Med.* 45:6.

———— 1961. Aldosteronism and hypertension. *Arch. Int. Med.* 107:813.

————, Cohen, E. L., and Rovner, D. R. 1964. Suppression of plasma renin activity in primary aldosteronism. *J.A.M.A.* 190:213.

————, Rovner, D. R., and Cohen, E. L. 1965. Normal and altered function of the renin-angiotensin-aldosterone system in man. *Ann. Intern. Med.* 63:266.

————, ————, ————, and Nesbit, R. M. 1966. Normokalemic primary aldosteronism: Its masquerade as essential hypertension. *J.A.M.A.* 195:21.

Cooper, D. Y., Touchstone, J. C., Roberts, J. M., Blakemore, W. S., and Rosenthal, O. 1958. Steroid formation by adrenal tissue from hypertensives. *J. Clin. Invest.* 37:1524.

Cope, C. L., Nicolis, G., and Fraser, B. 1961. Measurement of aldosterone secretion rate in man by the use of a metabolite. *Clin. Sci.* 21:367.

Cort, J. H. 1953. Effect of nervous stimulation of the arterio-venous oxygen and carbon dioxide differences across the kidney. *Nature* 171:784.

Costa, E. 1961. Renal concepts of the role of peripheral vs. central action of catecholamines in blood pressure regulation. In *Hypertension–Recent Advances: The Second Hahnemann Symposium on Hypertensive Disease,* edited by A. N. Brest and J. H. Moyer. Philadelphia: Lea & Febiger.

Cottier, P. T. 1960. Renal hemodynamics, water and electrolyte excretion in essential hypertension. In *Essential Hypertension,* edited by K. D. Bock and P. T. Cottier. Berlin: Springer.

Crane, M. G., and Harris, J. J. 1966. Desoxycorticosterone secretion rates in hyperadrenocorticism. *J. Clin. Endocrinol. Metab.* 26:1135.

Cranston, R. W., Chalmers, J. H., Taylor, H. L., Henschel, A., and Keys, A. 1949. Effect of a psychiatric interview on the blood pressure response to cold stimuli. *Fed. Proc.* 8:30.

Creditor, M. C., and Loschky, U. K. 1967. Plasma renin activity in hypertension. *Am. J. Med.* 43:371.

Crisp, A. H. 1963. Some current aspects of psychosomatic research. *Postgrad. Med. J.* 39:5.

Cross, B. A., and Green, J. D. 1959. Activity of single neurones in the hypothalamus: effect of osmotic and other stimuli. *J. Physiol.* (Lond.) 148:554.

Cruz-Coke, R. 1959. The hereditary factor in hypertension. *Acta Genet* (Basel) 9:207.

———— 1960. Environmental influences and arterial blood pressure. *Lancet* 2:885.

Dahl, L. K. 1959. Salt intake and salt need. *N. Engl. J. Med.* 258:1152.

———— 1960. Possible role of salt intake in the development of essential hypertension. In *Essential Hypertension,* edited by K. D. Bock and P. T. Cottier. Berlin: Springer.

———— and Love, R. A. 1957. Etiological role of sodium choloride in essential hypertension in humans. *J.A.M.A.* 164:397.

————, Heine, M., and Tassinari, L. 1962. Role of genetic factors in susceptibility to experimental hypertension due to chronic excess salt ingestion. *Nature* 194:480.

————, Knudsen, K. D., Heine, M., and Leitl, G. 1968. Effects of chronic excess salt ingestion: Modification of experimental hypertension in the rat by variations in the diet. *Circ. Res.* 22:11.

————, ————, and Iwai, J. 1969. Humoral transmission of hypertension: evidence from parabiosis. *Circ. Res.* Suppl. I, ad. 34/35:21.

————, Heine, M., and Thompson, K. 1972. Genetic influence of renal homografts on the blood pressure of rats from different strains. *Proc. Soc. Exp. Biol. Med.* 140:852.

Davies, M. H. 1970. Blood pressure and personality. *J. Psychosom. Res.* 14:89.

———— 1971. Is high blood pressure a psychosomatic disorder? *J. Chron. Dis.* 24:239.

Davis, J. O. 1961. A critical evaluation of the role of receptors in the control of aldosterone secretion and sodium excretion. *Prog. Cardiovasc. Dis.* 4:27.

———— 1974. Control of renin release. *Hosp. Pract.* 9:55.

————, Yankopoulos, N. A., Lieberman, F., Holman, J., and Bahn, R. C. 1960. The role of the anterior pituitary in the control of aldosterone secretion in experimental secondary hyperaldosteronism. *J. Clin. Invest.* 39:765.

————, Hartoft, P. M., Titus, E. O., and Carpenter, C. C. J. 1962. The role of the renin-angiotensin system in the control of aldosterone secretion. *J. Clin. Invest.* 41:378.

————, Urquhart, J., and Higgins, J. T., Jr. 1963. The effects of alterations of plasma sodium and potassium concentration on aldosterone secretion. *J. Clin. Invest.* 42:597.

————, Yankopoulos, N. A., Lieberman, F., Holman, J., and Bahn, R. C. 1970. The role of the anterior pituitary in the control of aldosterone secretion in experimental secondary hyperaldosteronism. *J. Clin. Invest.* 39:765.

Dawber, T. R., Kannel, W. B., Kagan, A., Donabedian, R. K., McNamara, P. M., and Pearson, G. 1967. Environmental factors in hypertension. In *The Epidemiology of Hypertension*, edited by J. Stamler, R. Stamler, and T. N. Pullman, New York: Grune & Stratton.

De Champlain, J. 1972. Hypertension and the sympathetic nervous system. In *Perspectives in Neuropharmacology*, edited by S. Snyder. Oxford: Oxford University Press.

De Champlain, J., Mueller, R. A., and Axelrod, J. 1969. Turnover and synthesis of norepinephrine in experimental hypertension in rats. *Circ. Res.* 25:285.

De Champlain, J., and van Amerigen, M. R. 1973. Role of sympathetic fibers and of adrenal medulla in the maintenance of cardiovascular homeostasis in normotensive and hypertensive rats. In *Frontiers in Catecholamine Research*, edited by E. Usdin and S. Snyder. Oxford: Pergamon.

DeJong, W. Lovenberg, W., and Sjoerdsma, A. 1972. Increased plasma renin activity in spontaneously hypertensive rats. *Proc. Soc. Exp. Biol. Med.* 139:1213.

Denton, D. 1961. Discussion of the lecture of J. O. Davis. *Recent Progr. Hormone Res.* 17:331.

DiPalma, J. R. 1961. Antihypertensive agents which affect catecholamine release. *Hypertension—Recent Advances: The Second Hahnemann Symposium on Hypertensive Disease*, edited by A. N. Brest and J. H. Moyer. Philadelphia: Lea & Febiger.

Doba, N. and Reis, D. J. 1973. Acute fulminating neurogenic hypertension produced by brain stem lesions in the rat. *Circ. Res.* 32:584.

————, and ————. 1974. Role of central and peripheral adrenergic mechanisms in neurogenic hypertension produced by brain stem lesion in rats. *Circ. Res.* 34:293.

Dock, W. 1940. Vasoconstriction in renal hypertension abolished by pithing. *Am. J. Physiol.* 130:1.

Dole, V. P., Dahl, L. K., Cotzias, G. C., Eder, H. A., and Krebs, M. E. 1951. Dietary treatment of hypertension. Clinical and metabolic studies of patients on the rice-fruit diet. *J. Clin. Invest.* 29:1189.

Dollery, C. T., Shakman, R., and Shillingford, J. 1959. Malignant hypertension and hypokalaemia cured by nephrectomy. *Brit. Med. J.* ii:1367.

Dontas, A. S. 1955. Effects of protoveratrine, serotonin and ATP on afferent and splanchnic nerve activity. *Circ. Res.* 3:363.

Douglas, W. W., and Ritchie, J. M. 1956. Cardiovascular reflexes produced by electrical excitation of non-medullated afferents in the vagus, carotid sinus and aortic nerves. *J. Physiol.* (Lond.) 134:167.

————, ————, and Schaumann, W. 1956. Depressor reflexes from medullated and non-medullated fibers in the rabbit's aortic nerve. *J. Physiol.* (Lond.) 132:187.

Downman, C. B. B. 1955. Skeletal muscle reflexes of splanchnic and intercostal nerve origin in acute spinal and decerebrate cats. *J. Neurophysiol.* 18:217.

Doyle, A. E., and Fraser, J. R. E. 1961. Essential hypertension and inheritance of vascular reactivity. *Lancet* ii:509.

Drury, D. R., and Schapiro, S. 1956. Renin tachyphylaxis and renal ischemia in the cat. *Am. J. Physiol.* 187:520.

Dunbar, H. F. 1943. *Psychosomatic Diagnosis.* New York: Hoeber.

Dykman, R. A., and Gantt, W. H. 1960. Experimental psychogenic hypertension: blood pressure changes conditioned to painful stimuli (Schizokinesis). *Bull. Johns Hopkins Hosp.* 107:72.

Ead, H. W., Green, J. H., and Neil, E. 1952. A comparison of the effects of pulsatile and non-pulsatile flow through the carotid sinus on the reflexogenic activity of the sinus baroreceptors in the cat. *J. Physiol.* (Lond.) 119:509.

Ehrlich, E. N. 1968. Aldosterone, the adrenal cortex, and hypertension. *Annu. Rev. Med.* 19:373.

————, Lugibihl, K., Laves, M., and Janulis, M. 1966. Reciprocal variations in urinary cortisol and aldosterone in response to increased salt intake in humans. *J. Clin. Endocrinol. Metab.* 26:1160.

————, ————, Taylor, C., and Janulis, M. 1967. Reciprocal variations in urinary cortisol and aldosterone in response to the sodium-depleting influence of hydrochlorothiazide and ethacrynic acid in humans. *J. Clin. Endocrinol. Metab.* 27:836.

Ehrstrom, M. D. 1945. Psychogene Blutdruckssteigerung in Kriegshypertonien. *Acta Med. Scand.* 122:546.

Eich, R. H., Cuddy, R. P. Smulyan, H., and Lyons, R. H. 1966. Haemodynamics in labile hypertension. *Circulation* 34:299.

Eichna, L. W., and McQuarrie, D. G. 1960. Proceedings of a Symposium on Central Nervous System Control of Circulation. *Physiol. Rev.* Suppl. 4, 40.

Eide, I., Løyning, E., and Kiil, F. 1973. Evidence for hemodynamic autoregulation of renin release. *Circ. Res.* 32:237.

Eisenstein, A. B., and Hartroft, P. M. 1956. Sodium deficiency and adrenocortical hormone secretion. *J. Lab. Clin. Med.* 48:802.

Eliasson, S., Lindgren, P., and Uvnäs, B. 1952. Representation in the hypothalamus and the motor cortex in the dog of the sympathetic vasodilator outflow to the skeletal muscles. *Acta Physiol. Scand.* 27:18.

————, ————, and ———— 1954. The hypothalamus, a relay station of the sympathetic vasodilator tract. *Acta Physiol. Scand.* 31:290.

Ellis, M. E., and Grollman, A. 1949. The antidiuretic hormone in the urine in experimental and clinical hypertension. *Endocrinology* 44:415.

Elmadjian, F., Hope, J. M., and Lamson, E. T. 1957. Excretion of epinephrine and norepinephrine in various emotional states. *J. Clin. Endocrinol. Metab.* 17:608.

Emanuel, D., Scott, J. B., and Haddy, F. J. 1959. Effect of potassium upon small and large blood vessels of the dog forelimb. *Am. J. Physiol.* 197:637.

Engel, B. T., and Bickford, A. F. 1961. Response specificity. *Arch. Gen. Psychiatry* 5:82.

Engelman, K., Portnoy, B., and Sjoerdsma, A. 1970. Plasma catecholamine concentrations in patients with hypertension. *Circ. Res.* 26–27(Suppl. 1):141.

Epstein, A. N., Fitzimmons, J. T., and Rolls, B. J. 1970. Drinking induced by injection of angiotensin into the brain of the rat. *J. Physiol.* (Lond.) 210:457.

Evans, G. 1920. A contribution to the study of arterial-sclerosis with special reference to its relation to chronic renal disease. *Q. J. Med.* 14:215.

Evans, W. 1957. Hypertonia or uneventful high blood pressure. *Lancet* ii:53.

Fallis, N., Lasagna, L., and Tetreault, L. 1962. Gustatory thresholds in patients with hypertension. *Nature* 196:74.

Farnsworth, E. B. 1946. Renal reabsorption of chloride and phosphate in normal subjects and in patients with essential hypertension. *J. Clin. Invest.* 25:897.

Farrell, G. 1958. Regulation of aldosterone secretion. *Physiol. Rev.* 38:709.

———— 1959a. Glomerulotropic activity of an acetone extract of pineal tissue. *Endocrinology* 65:239.

———— 1959b. The physiological factors which influence the secretion of aldosterone. *Recent Progr. Hormone Res.* 15:275.

———— 1963. Discussion of the lecture by J. R. Blair-West. *Recent Prog. Horm. Res.* 19:367.

Farris, E. J., Yeakel, E. H., and Medoff, H. S. 1945. Development of hypertension in emotional gray Norwegian rats after airblasting. *Am. J. Physiol.* 144:331.

Feigl, E. O., Peterson, L. H., and Jones, A. W. 1963. Mechanical and chemical properties of arteries in experimental hypertension. *J. Clin. Invest.* 42:1640.

Fernandez De Molina, A., and Hunsperger, R. W. 1959. Central representation of affective reactions in forebrain and brain stem: Electrical stimulation of amygdala, stria terminalis, and adjacent structures. *J. Physiol.* (Lond.) 145:251.

────── and ────── 1962. Organization of the subcortical system governing defence and flight reactions in the cat. *J. Physiol.* (Lond.) 160:200.

Ferrario, C. M., Dickinson, C. J., Gildenberg, P. L., and McCubbin, J. W. 1969. Central vasomotor stimulation by angiotensin. *Fed. Proc.* 28:394.

──────, Gildenberg, P. L., and McCubbin, J. W. 1972. Cardiovascular effects of angiotensin mediated by the central nervous system. *Circ. Res.* 30:257.

──────, Page, I. H., and McCubbin, J. W. 1970. Increased cardiac output as a contributing factor in experimental renal hypertension in dogs. *Circ. Res.* 27:799.

Figar, S. 1965. Conditional circulatory responses in man and animals. In *Handbook of Physiology,* sect. 2, vol. 3, Washington, D.C.: American Physiological Society.

Finch, L., Haeusler, G., and Thoenen, H. 1972. Failure to induce experimental hypertension in rats after intraventricular injection of 6-hydroxydopamine. *Br. J. Pharmacol.* 44:356.

Finkielman, S., Worcel, M., and Agrest, A. 1965. Hemodynamic patterns in essential hypertension. *Circulation* 31:356.

Finnerty, F. A., Jr., Davidov, M., and Kakaviatos, N. 1968. Relation of sodium balance to arterial pressure during drug-induced saluresis. *Circulation* 37:175.

Fischer, H. K. 1961. Hypertension and the psyche. In *Hypertension—Recent Advances: The Second Hahnemann Symposium on Hypertensive Disease,* edited by A. N. Brest and J. H. Moyer. Philadelphia: Lea & Febiger.

Floyer, M. A. 1955. Further studies on the mechanism of experimental hypertension in the rat. *Clin. Sci.* 14:163.

Flynn, J. T., Kennedy, M. A. K., and Wolf, S. 1950. Essential hypertension in one of identical twins. An experimental study of cardiovascular reactions in the Y twins. *Res. Publ. Assoc. Nerv. Ment. Dis.* 29:954.

Folkow, B. 1952. Impulse frequency in sympathetic vasomotor fibres correlated to release and elimination of transmitter. *Acta Physiol. Scand.* 25:49.

────── 1971. The haemodynamic consequences of adaptive structural changes of the resistance vessels in hypertension. *Clin. Sci.* 41:1.

──────, Strom, G., and Uvnäs, B. 1950. Do dorsal root fibres convey centrally induced vasodilator impulses? *Acta Physiol. Scand.* 21:145.

────── and Uvnäs, B. 1948. The chemical tramission of vasoconstrictor impulses to the hind limbs and the splanchnic region of the cat. *Acta Physiol. Scand.* 15:365.

────── and ────── 1950. Do adrenergic vasodilator nerves exist? *Acta Physiol. Scand.* 20:329.

────── and Rubinstein, E. H. 1966. Cardiovascular effects of acute and chronic stimulations of the hypothalamic defence area in the rat. *Acta Physiol. Scand.* 68:48.

──────, Löfving, B., and Mellander, S. 1956. Quantitative aspects of sympathetic neurohormonal control of heart rate. *Acta Physiol. Scand.* 37:363.

──────, Mellander, S., and Öberg, B. 1961. The range of effect of the sympathetic vasodilator fibres with regard to consecutive sections of the muscle vessels. *Acta Physiol. Scand.* 53:7.

──────, Hedner, P., Lisander, B., and Rubinstein, E. H. 1965. Release of cortisol upon stimulation of the hypothalamic defence area in cats. A symposium on stress. *Försvarsmed. Tidskrift.*

──────, Hallbäck, M., Lundren, Y., and Weiss, L. 1970. Structurally based increase of flow resistance in spontaneously hypertensive rats. *Acta Physiol. Scand.* 79:373.

──────, ──────, ──────, Sivertsson, R., and Weiss, L. 1973. Importance of adaptive changes in vascular design for establishment of primary hypertension, studied in man and in spontaneously hypertensive rats. *Circ. Res.* 32(Suppl. I):I–2.

Forsyth, R. P. 1968. Blood pressure and avoidance conditioning. *Psychosom. Med.* 30:125.

————— 1969. Blood pressure responses to long-term avoidance schedules in the restrained rhesus monkey. *Psychosom. Med.* 31:300.

Franco-Browder, S., Masson, G. M. C., and Corcoran, A. C. 1958. Pharmacologic characterization of reserpine responses in rats pretreated with iproniazid. *Proc. Soc. Exp. Biol. Med.* 97:778.

Freis, E. D. 1960. Hemodynamics of hypertension. *Physiol. Rev.* 40:27.

—————, Wanko, A., Wilson, I. M., and Parrish, A. E. 1958. Treatment of essential hypertension with chlorothiazide (diuril). *J.A.M.A.* 166:137.

Friedman, E. H., Hellerstein, H. K., Eastwood, G. L., and Jones, S. E. 1968. Behavior patterns and serum cholesterol in two groups of normal males. *Am. J. Med. Sci.* 255:237.

Friedman, M., and Kasanin, J. S. 1943. Hypertension in only one of identical twins: report of a case with consideration of psychosomatic factors. *Arch. Intern. Med.* 72:767.

————— and Rosenman, R. H. 1959. Association of specific overt behavior pattern with blood and cardiovascular findings. *J.A.M.A.* 169:1286.

Friedman, R., and Dahl, L. K. 1975. The effect of chronic conflict on the blood pressure of rats with a genetic susceptibility to experimental hypertension. *Psychosom. Med.* 37:402.

Fritz, I., and Levine, R. 1951. Action of adrenal cortical steroids and norepinephrine on vascular responses of stress in adrenalectomized rats. *Am. J. Physiol.* 165:456.

Frohlich, E. D., Tarazi, R. C., and Dustan, H. P. 1969. Re-examination of the hemodynamics of hypertension. *Am. J. Med. Sci.* 257:9.

—————, Kozul, V. J., Tarazi, K. C., and Dustan, H. P. 1970. Physiological comparison of labile and essential hypertension. *Circ. Res.* 26–27:1.

Froňková, K., Ehrlich, V., and Šlégr, L. 1957. Die Kreislaufänderung beim Hunde während des bedingten und unbedingten Nährungsreflexes und seiner Hemmung. *Pflügers Arch.* 236:704.

—————, —————, and ————— 1959. Changes in resting blood pressure values during elaboration of conditioned reflexes and their active inhibition. *Physiol. Bohemoslov.* 8:40.

Fukuda, T. 1951. L'hypertension par le sel chez les lapins et ses relations avec la glande surrénale. *Union Méd. Can.* 80:1278.

Fukyama, K. 1973. Central modulation of baroreceptor reflex by angiotensin. *Japon. Heart J.* 14:135.

Funder, J. W., Blair-West, J. R., Cain, M. C., Catt, K. J., Coghlan, J. P., Denton, D. A., Nelson, J. F., Scoggins, B. A., and Wright, R. D. 1970. Circulatory and humoral changes in the reversal of renovascular hypertension in sheep by unclipping the renal artery. *Circ. Res.* 27:249.

Funkenstein, D. H., King, S. H., and Drolette, M. E. 1957. *The Mastery of Stress.* Cambridge, Mass.: Harvard University Press.

Fuxe, K. 1965. Distribution of monoamine terminals in the central nervous system. *Acta Physiol. Scand.* 64(Suppl. 247):38.

Gampel, M. B., Slome, C., Scotch, N., and Abramson, J. H. 1962. Urbanization and hypertension among Zulu adults. *J. Chronic Dis.* 15:67.

Ganong, W. F. 1972. Effects of sympathetic activity and ACTH on renin and aldosterone secretion. In *Hypertension 1972*, edited by J. Genest and E. Koiw. Berlin: Springer.

Ganten, D., Hutchinson, J. S., Hackenthal, E., Schelling, P., Rosas, B. P., and Genest, J. 1974. Intrinsic brain iso-renin-angiotensin system. (ISO-RAS) and hypertension in rats. *Clin. Sci.* (Suppl.)

Ganten, D., Marquez-Julio, A., Granger, P., Hayduk, K., Karsunsky, K. P., Boucher, R., and Genest, J. 1971. Renin in dog brain. *Am. J. Physiol.* 221:1733.

Gantt, W. H. 1935. Effect of alcohol on cortical and subcortical activity measured by conditioned reflex method. *Bull. Johns Hopkins Hosp.* 56:61.

————— 1958. *Physiological Basis of Psychiatry.* Springfield, Ill.: Charles C Thomas.

———— 1960. Cardiovascular component of the conditioned reflex to pain, food and other stimuli. *Physiol. Rev.* 40(Suppl. 4):266.

Garst, J. B., Shumway, N. P., Schwartz, H., and Farrel, G. L. 1960. Aldosterone excretion in essential hypertension. *J. Clin. Endocrinol. Metab.* 20:1351.

Gauer, O. H., and Henry, J. P. 1963. Circulatory basis of fluid volume control. *Physiol. Rev.* 43:423.

Gavlichek, V. A. 1952. Changes of the blood pressure level during various functional states of the cortex in dogs. *Vyschey Nervnoy Dejatelmosty* 2:742.

Gearing, F. R., Clark, E. G., Perera, G. A., and Schweitzer, M. D. 1962. Hypertension among relatives of hypertensives. *Am. J. Public Health* 52:2058.

Gelshteyn, E. M. 1943. Clinical characteristics of hypertensive disease under wartime conditions. *Klin. Med.* (Mosk.) 21:10.

Genest, J. 1961. Angiotensin, aldosterone and human arterial hypertension. *Can. Med. Assoc. J.* 84:403.

———— 1974. Basic mechanisms in benign essential hypertension. *Hosp. Pract.* 9:97.

————, Koiw, E., Nowaczynski, W., and Sandor, T. 1960. Study of a large steroid spectrum in normal subjects and hypertensive patients. *Acta Endocrinol.* (Kbh.) 35:413.

————, Boucher, R., De Champlain, J., Veyrat, R., Chretien, M., Birow, P., Tremblay, G., Roy, P., and Cartier, P. 1964. Studies on the renin-angiotensin system in hypertensive patients. *Can. Med. Assoc. J.* 90:263.

————, ————, Kuchel, O., and Nowaczynski, W. 1973. Renin in hypertension: how important as a risk factor? *Can. Med. Assoc. J.* 109:475.

Giese, J. 1964. Acute hypertensive vascular disease: I. Relation between blood pressure changes and vascular lesions in different forms of actue hypertension. *Acta Pathol. Microbiol. Scand.* 62:481.

Gildenberg, P. L. 1971. Site of angiotensin vasopressor activity in the brain stem. *Fed. Proc.* 30:432.

Gill, J. R., Jr., Mason, D. T., and Bartter, F. C. 1964. Adrenergic nervous system in sodium metabolism: Effects of guanethidine and sodium-retaining steroids in normal man. *J. Clin. Invest.* 43:177.

Girling, F. 1952. Vasomotor effects of electrical stimulation. *Am. J. Physiol.* 170:131.

Gitlow, S. E., Mendlowitz, M., Kruk-Wilk, E., Wilk, S., Wolf, R. L., and Naftchi, N. E. 1964. Plasma clearance of dl-H³-norepinephrine in normal human subjects and patients with essential hypertension. *J. Clin. Invest.* 43:2009.

Glock, C. Y., and Lennard, H. L. 1957. Studies in hypertension. V. Psychologic factors in hypertension: An interpretative review. *J. Chronic Dis.* 5:174.

————, Vought, R. L., Clark, E. G., and Schweitzer, M. D. 1957. Studies in hypertension. II. Variability of daily blood pressure measurements in the same individuals over a three-week period. *J. Chronic Dis.* 4:469.

Glowinski, J., and Baldessarini, R. J. 1966. Metabolism of norepinephrine in the central nervous system. *Pharmacol. Rev.* 18:1201.

Goldblatt, H. 1947. Renal origin of hypertension. *Physiol. Rev.* 27:120.

Goldenberg, M., Pines, K. L., Baldwin, E. F., Greene, D. G., and Roh, C. E. 1948. Hemodynamic response of man to norepinephrine and epinephrine and its relation to the problem of hypertension. *Am. J. Med.* 5:792.

Goldring, E., Chasis, H., Schneiner, G. E., and Smith, H. W. 1956. Reassurance in the management of benign hypertensive disease. *Circulation* 14:260.

Gomez, A., Hoobler, S. W., and Blaquier, P. 1960. Effect of addition and removal of a kidney transplant in renal and adrenocortical hypertensive rats. *Circ. Res.* 8:464.

100

Goodall, M., and Bogdonoff, M. 1961. Essential hypertension with elevated noradrenaline excretion. *Am. Heart J.* 61:640.

Gordon, R. D., Spector, S., Sjoerdsma, A., and Udenfriend, S. 1966. Increased synthesis of norepinephrine and epinephrine in the intact rat during exercise and exposure to cold. *J. Pharmacol. Exp. Ther.* 153:440.

————, Kuchel, O., Liddle, G. W., and Island, D. W. 1967. Role of the sympathetic nervous system in regulating renin and aldosterone production in man. *J. Clin. Invest.* 46:599.

Gottschalk, L., and Hambidge, G. 1955. Verbal behavior analysis: A systematic approach to the problem of quantifying psychologic processes. *J. Project. Techn.* 19:387.

Grace, W. J., and Graham, D. T. 1952. Relationship of specific attitudes and emotions to certain bodily diseases. *Psychosom. Med.* 14:243.

Graham, D. T., Kabler, J. D., and Graham, F. K. 1960. Experimental production of predicted physiological differences by suggestion of attitude. *Psychosom. Med.* 22:321.

————, ————, and ———— 1962a. Physiological response to the suggestion of attitudes specific for hives and hypertension. *Psychosom. Med.* 24:159.

————, Lundy, R. M., Benjamin, L. S., Kabler, J. D., Lewis, W. C., Kunish, N. O., and Graham, F. K. 1962b. Specific attitudes in initial interviews with patients having different "psychosomatic" diseases. *Psychosom. Med.* 24:257.

Graham, J. D. P. 1945. High blood pressure after battle. *Lancet* i:239.

Green, D. M., and Ellis, E. J. 1954. Sodium-output-blood pressure relationships and their modification by treatment. *Circulation* 10:536.

Griffith, L. S. C., and Schwartz, S. I. 1963. Electrical stimulation of the carotid sinus nerve in normotensive and renal hypertensive dogs. *Circulation* 28:730.

———— and ———— 1964. Reversal of renal hypertension by electrical stimulation of the carotid sinus nerve. *Surgery* 56:232.

Grollman, A. 1960. Therapeutic aspects of salt restriction. In *Essential Hypertension,* edited by K. D. Bock and P. T. Cottier. Berlin: Springer.

————, Harrison, T. R., and Williams, J. R., Jr. 1940. The effect of various steroid derivatives on the blood pressure of the rat. *J. Pharmacol. Exp. Ther.* 69:149.

————, Muirhead, E. E., and Vanatta, J. 1949. Role of the kidney in the pathogenesis of hypertension as determined by a study of the effects of bilateral nephrectomy and other experimental procedures on the blood pressure of the dog. *Am. J. Physiol.* 157:21.

Gross, F. 1960. Adrenocortical function and renal pressor mechanisms in experimental hypertension. In *Essential Hypertension,* edited by K. D. Bock and P. T. Cottier. Berlin: Springer.

———— 1971. The renin-angiotensin system and hypertension. *Ann. Intern. Med.* 75:777.

———— and Lichtlen, P. 1958. Pressor substances in kidneys of renal hypertensive rats with and without adrenals. *Proc. Soc. Exp. Biol. Med.* 98:341.

———— and Sulser, F. 1956. Wirkungsverstärkerung von Renin und Nierenextrakt an der nierenlosen Ratte. *Naunyn-Schmiederbergs Arch. Pharmacol.* 229:338.

Groves, L. K., and Effler, D. B. 1960. Problems in surgical management of coarctation of the aorta. *J. Thorac. Cardiovasc. Surg.* 39:60.

Guillemin, R., Hearn, W. R., Cheek, W. R., and Householder, D. E. 1957. Control of corticotrophin release: further studies with *in vitro* methods. *Endocrinology* 60:488.

Gunnels, J. C., Jr., Grim, C. E., Robinson, R. R., Wildemann, N. M. 1967. Plasma renin activity in healthy subjects and patients with hypertension. Preliminary experience with a quantitative bioassay. *Arch. Int. Med.* 119:232.

Gutmann, F. D., Tagawa, H., Haber, E., and Barger, A. C. 1973. Renal arterial pressure, renin secretion, and blood pressure control in trained dogs. *Am. J. Physiol.* 224:66.

Gutmann, M. C., and Benson, H. 1971. Interaction of environmental factors and systemic arterial pressure. *Medicine* 50:543.

Guyton, A. C., and Coleman, T. G. 1969. Quantitative analysis of the pathophysiology of hypertension. *Circ. Res.* 24 (Suppl.):I–1.

Haeusler, G., Finch, L., and Thoenen, H. 1972a. Central adrenergic neurons and the initiation and development of experimental hypertension. *Experientia* 28:1200.

———, Gerold, J., and Thoenen, T. 1972b. Cardiovascular effects of 6-hydroxydopamine injected into a lateral brain ventricle of the rat. *Naunyn-Schmiedebergs Arch. Pharmacol.* 274:211.

Hambling, J. 1951. Emotions and symptoms of essential hypertension. *Br. J. Med. Psychol.* 24:242.

——— 1952. Psychosomatic aspects of essential hypertension. *Br. J. Med. Psychol.* 25:39.

Hamet, P., Kuchel, O., Cuche, J. L., Boucher, R., and Genest, J. 1973a. Effects of propranolol on cyclic AMP excretion and plasma renin activity in labile essential hypertension. *Can. Med. Assoc. J.* 109:1099.

———, ———, and Genest, J. 1973b. Effect of upright posture and isoproterenol infusion on cyclic adenosine monophosphate excretion in control subjects and patients with labile hypertension. *J. Clin. Endocrinol.* 36:218.

Hamilton, J. A. 1942. Psychophysiology of blood pressure—I. Personality and behavior ratings. *Psychosom. Med.* 4:125.

Hamilton, M., Pickering, G. W., Roberts, J. A. F., and Sowry, G. S. C. 1954. The etiology of essential hypertension. *Clin. Sci. Mol. Med.* 13:273.

———, ———, ———, and ——— 1963. Arterial pressures of relatives of patients with secondary and malignant hypertension. *Clin. Sci. Mol. Med.* 24:91.

Handley, C. A., and Moyer, J. H. 1954. Changes in sodium and water excretion by vaso-active and by ganglionic and adrenergic blocking agents. *Am. J. Physiol.* 178:309.

Harburg, E., Julius, S., McGinn, N. F., McLeod, J., and Hoobler, S. W. 1964. Personality traits and behavioral patterns associated with systolic blood pressure levels in college males. *J. Chronic Dis.* 17:405.

———, McGinn, N. F., and Wigle, J. B. 1965. Recalled treatment by parents among college males and blood pressure levels vs. variability. *J. Psychosom. Res.* 9:173.

———, Erfurt, J. C., Hauenstein, L. S., Chape, C., Schull, W. J., and Schork, M. A. 1973. Socio-ecological stress, suppressed hostility, skin color, and black-white male blood pressure: Detroit. *Psychosom. Med.* 35:276.

Hardyck, C., and Singer, M. T. 1962. Transient changes in affect and blood pressure. *Arch. Gen. Psychiatry* 7:15.

Harris, G. W. 1947. The innervation and actions of the neurohypophysis; an investigation using the method of remote-control stimulation. *Philos. Trans. R. Soc. Lond.* [*Biol.*] 232b:385.

Harris, R. E., and Singer, M. T. 1968. Interaction of personality and stress in the pathogenesis of essential hypertension. In *Hypertension. Neural Control of Arterial Pressure.* Volume 16 in *Proceedings of the Council for High Blood Pressure Research.* New York: American Heart Association.

———, Sokolow, M., Carpenter, L. G., Freedman, M., and Hunt, S. P. 1953. Response to psychologic stress in persons who are potentially hypertensive. *Circulation* 7:874.

Harris, W. S., Schoenfeld, C. D., Gwynne, P. H., Weissler, A. M., and Warren, J. V. 1965. Circulatory and humoral responses to fear and anger. *J. Lab. Clin. Med.* 64:867.

Hayward, J. N., and Smith, W. K. 1962. The role of mesencephalic tegmental structures in the regulation of neurohypophysial function. *Fed. Proc.* 21:354.

Helmer, O. M. 1964. Renin activity in blood from patients with hypertension. *Can. Med. Assoc. J.* 90:221.

Henning, M. 1969. Noradrenaline turnover in renal hypertensive rats. *J. Pharm. Pharmacol.* 21:1969.

Henry, J. P., and Cassel, J. C. 1969. Psychosocial factors in essential hypertension. Recent epidemiologic and animal experimental evidence. *Am. J. Epidemiol.* 90:171.

———, Meehan, J. P., and Stephens, P. M. 1967. The use of psychosocial stimuli to induce prolonged systolic hypertension in mice. *Psychosom. Med.* 29:408.

———, Stephens, P. M., Axelrod, J., and Mueller, R. A. 1971a. Effect of psychosocial stimulation on the enzymes involved in the biosynthesis and metabolism of noradrenaline and adrenaline. *Psychosom. Med.* 33:227.

———, Ely, D. L., and Stephens, P. M. 1971b. Role of the autonomic system in social adaptation and stress. *Proc. Int. Union Physiol. Sci.* 8:50.

Herd, J. A., Morse, W. H., Kelleher, R. T., and Jones, J. G. 1969. Arterial hypertension in the squirrel monkey during behavioral experiments. *Am. J. Physiol.* 217:24.

Hering, H. E. 1923. Das Carotisdruckversuch. *Münch. Med. Wochenschr.* 42:1

Hess, W. 1949. *Das Zwischenhirn*. Basel: Schwabe.

Heyden, S., Bartel, A. G., Hames, C. G., and McDonough, J. R. 1969. Elevated blood pressure levels in adolescents, Evans County, Georgia: 7-year follow-up of 30 patients and 30 controls. *J.A.M.A.* 209:1683.

Heymans, C., and Neil, E. 1958. *Reflexogenic Areas of the Cardiovascular System*. Boston: Little, Brown.

Hickler, R. B., Lauler, D. P., Saravis, C. A., and Thorn, G. W. 1964. Characterization of a vasodepressor lipid of the renal medulla. *Trans. Assoc. Am. Physicians* 77:196.

Hill, L. B. 1935. A psychoanalytic observation on essential hypertension. *Psychoanal. Rev.* 22:60.

Hillarp, N.-A., Fuxe, K., and Dahlstrom, A. 1966. Demonstration and mapping of central neurons containing dopamine, noradrenaline, and 5-hydroxytryptamine and their reactions to psychopharmacological agents. *Pharmacol. Rev.* 18:727.

Hines, E. A., Jr. 1940. Range of normal blood pressure and subsequent development of hypertension: A follow-up study of 1522 patients. *J.A.M.A.* 115:271.

———, McIlhaney, M. L., and Gage, R. P. 1957. A study of twins with normal blood pressures and with hypertension. *Trans. Assoc. Am. Physicians* 70:282.

Hoff, E. C., and Green, H. D. 1936. Cardiovascular reactions induced by electrical stimulation of cerebral cortex. *Am. J. Physiol.* 117:411.

———, Kell, J. F., Jr., Hastings, N., Gray, E. N., and Scholes, D. M. 1951. Vasomotor, cellular and functional changes produced in kidney by brain stimulation. *J. Neurophysiol.* 14:317.

Hoff, H. E., Breckenridge, C. G., and Spencer, W. A. 1952. Suprasegmental integration of cardiac innervation. *Am. J. Physiol.* 171:178.

Hokanson, J. E. 1961a. The effects of frustration and anxiety on overt aggression. *J. Abnorm. Psychol.* 62:346.

——— 1961b. Vascular and psychogalvanic effects of experimentally aroused anger. *J. Pers.* 29:30.

Hollander, W., and Wilkins, R. W. 1957. Chlorothiazide: A new type of drug for the treatment of arterial hypertension. *Boston Med. Q.* 8:69.

Holloway, E. T., Seidel, C. L., and Bohr, D. F. 1973. Altered dependence on calcium of vascular smooth muscle from animals with experimental hypertension. *Hypertension, 1972. Second International Symposium on the Renin-Angiotensin-Aldosterone-Sodium System in Hypertension*, Mont Gabriel, Quebec. Berlin: Springer.

Holtz, P., Credner, K., and Kroneberg, G. 1947. Über das sympathicomimetische pressorische des Harns ("Urosympathin"). *Naunyn-Schmiedebergs Arch. Pharmacol.* 204:228.

Holzbauer, M., and Vogt, M. 1956. Depression by reserpine of the noradrenaline concentration in the hypothalamus of the cat. *J. Neurochem.* 1:8.

Hoobler, S. W. 1961. Current concepts of the mechanism of essential hypertension. In *Hypertension—Recent Advances: The Second Hahnemann Symposium on Hypertensive Disease*, edited by A. N. Brest and J. H. Moyer. Philadelphia: Lea & Febiger.

Horwitz, D., Alexander, R. W., Lovenberg, W., and Keiser, H. R. 1973. Human serum dopamine—β-hydroxylase: relationship to hypertension and sympathetic activity. *Circ. Res.* 32:594.

Humphrey, D. R. 1967. Neuronal activity in the medulla oblongata of cat evoked by stimulation of the carotid sinus nerve. In *Baroreceptors and Hypertension,* edited by P. Kezdi. New York: Pergamon.

Hunsperger, R. W. 1956. Affectreaktione auf elektrische Reizung im Hirnstamm der Katze. *Helv. Physiol. Acta* 14:7.

Ikoma, T. 1965. Studies on catechols with reference to hypertension (chap. I). *Jpn. Circ. J.* 29:1269.

Innes, G., Miller, W. M., and Valentine, M. 1959. Emotion and blood pressure. *J. Ment. Sci.* 105:840.

Iwai, J., Dahl, L. K., and Knudsen, K. D. 1973. Genetic influence on the renin-angiotensin system. Low renin activities in hypertension-prone rats. *Circ. Res.* 32:678.

Jaffe, D., Dahl, L. K., Sutherland, L., and Barker, D. 1969. Effects of chronic excess salt ingestion: Morphological findings in kidneys of rats with differing genetic susceptibility to hypertension. *Fed. Proc.* 28:422.

Jarrot, B., McQueen, A., and Louis, W. J. 1975. Serotonin levels in vascular tissue and the effects of a serotonin synthesis inhibitor on blood pressure in rats. *Clin. Exp. Pharmacol. Physiol.* 2:201.

Jenkins, C. D., Rosenman, R. H., and Friedman, M. 1967. Development of an objective psychological test for the determination of the coronary-prone behavior pattern in employed men. *J. Chronic Dis.* 20:371.

Johnson, B. C., and Remington, R. D. 1961. A sampling study of blood pressure levels in white and Negro residents of Nassau, Bahamas. *J. Chronic Dis.* 13:39.

———, Epstein, F. H., and Kjelsberg, M. O. 1965. Distributions and familial studies of blood pressure and serum cholesterol levels in a rural community—Tecumseh, Michigan. *J. Chronic Dis.* 18:147.

Jones, S. H., Younghusband, O. Z., and Evans, J. A. 1948. Human parabiotic pygopagus twins with essential hypertension. *J.A.M.A.* 138:642.

Jose, A., Crout, J. R., and Kaplan, N. M. 1970. Suppressed plasma renin activity in essential hypertension: roles of plasma volume, blood pressure and sympathetic nervous system. *Ann. Intern. Med.* 72:9.

Jost, H., Ruilmann, C. J., Hill, T. S., and Gulo, M. J. 1952. Studies in hypertension II: central and autonomic nervous system reactions of hypertensive individuals to simple physical and psychologic stress situations. *J. Nerv. Ment. Dis.* 115:152.

Joy, M. D., and Lowe, R. D. 1970. The site of cardiovascular action of angiotensin II in the brain. *Clin. Sci. Mol. Med.* 39:327.

Juan, P. 1963. Epiphyse, 5-hydroxytryptamine et corticoidogenese in vitro. *Ann. Endocrinol.* (Paris) 24:365.

Julius, S., and Conway, J. 1968. Hemodynamic studies in patients with borderline blood pressure elevation. *Circulation* 38:282.

——— and Schork, M. A. 1971. Borderline hypertension—a critical review. *J. Chronic Dis.* 23:723.

———, Harburg, E., McGinn, N. F., Keyes, J., and Hoobler, S. W. 1964. Relation between casual blood pressure readings in youth and at age 40: A retrospective study. *J. Chronic Dis.* 17:397.

———, Sannerstedt, R., and Conway, J. 1968. Hemodynamic effects of propranolol in borderline hypertension. *Circulation* 37 (Suppl. 6):109.

Kaada, B. R. 1951. Somatomotor, autonomic and electrocorticographic responses to electrical stimulation of "rhinencephalic" and other structures in primate, cat and dog. *Acta Physiol. Scand.* 83 (Suppl. 24):1.

———, Pribram, K. H., and Epstein, J. A. 1949. Respiratory and vascular responses in monkeys from temporal pole, insula, oribal surface and angulate gyrus. *J. Neurophysiol.* 12:347.

Kagan, A., Gordon, T., Kannel, W. B., and Dawber, T. R. 1958. Blood pressure and its relation to coronary heart disease in the Framingham study. *Hypertension* 7:53.

Kalis, B. L., Harris, R. E., Bennett, L. F., and Sokolow, M. 1961. Personality and life history factors in persons who are potentially hypertensive. *J. Nerv. Ment. Dis.* 132:457.

Kaminskiy, S. D. 1951. Role of central mechanisms in development of hypertension. *Klin. Med.* (Mosk.) 29:22.

Kandel, E. R. 1964. Electrical properties of hypothalamic neuroendocrine cells. *J. Gen. Physiol.* 47:691.

Kaneko, Y., Ikeda, T., Takeda, T., and Ueda, H. 1967. Renin release during acute reduction of arterial pressure in normotensive subjects and patients with renovascular hypertension. *J. Clin. Invest.* 46:705.

———, ———, ———, Inoue, G., Tagawa, H., and Ueda, H. 1968. Renin release in patients with benign essential hypertension. *Circulation* 38:353.

Kannel, W. B., Schwartz, M. J., and McNamara, P. M. 1969. Blood pressure and risk of coronary heart disease: The Framingham study. *Dis. Chest* 56:43.

Kaplan, S. M., Gottschalk, L. A., Magliocco, B., Rohovit, D., and Ross, W. D. 1960. Hostility in verbal productions and hypnotic "dreams" of hypertensive patients (comparisons between hypertensive and normotensive groups and within hypertensive individuals). *Psychosom. Med.* 22:320.

Karczmar, A. G., and Scudder, C. L. 1967. Behavioral responses to drugs and brain catecholamine levels in mice of different strains and genera. *Fed. Proc.* 26:1186.

Karli, P. 1969. Rat-mouse interspecific aggressive behavior and its manipulation by brain ablations and by brain stimulation. In *Biology of Aggressive Behavior,* edited by S. Garattini and E. B. Sigg. Amsterdam: Excerpta Medica.

Keith, R. L., Lown, B., and Stare, F. J. 1965. Coronary heart disease and behavior patterns. *Psychosom. Med.* 27:424.

Kezdi, P. 1962. Mechanism of the carotid sinus in experimental hypertension. *Circ. Res.* 11:145.

——— (ed.) 1967. *Baroreceptors and Hypertension.* New York: Pergamon.

——— and Wennemark, J. R. 1958. Baroreceptor and sympathetic activity in experimental renal hypertension in the dog. *Circulation* 17:785.

King, S. E., and Baldwin, D. S. 1956. Production of renal ischemia and proteinuria in man by the adrenal medullary hormones. *Am. J. Med.* 20:217.

Kirkendall, W. M., Fitz, A., and Armstrong, M. L. 1964. Hypokalemia and the diagnosis of hypertension. *Dis. Chest* 45:337.

Knowlton, A. I. 1960. Comparison of effect of desoxycorticosterone acetate and cortisone acetate on rat skeletal muscle electrolytes. *Proc. Soc. Exp. Biol. Med.* 104:13.

———, Loeb, E. N., Stoerk, H. C., and Seegal, B. C. 1947. Desoxycorticosterone acetate. The potentiation of its activity by sodium chloride. *J. Exp. Med.* 85:187.

Koch, E. 1931. *Die reflektorische Selbsteuerung des Kreislaufes.* Leipzig: Steinkopf.

Kogel, J. E., and Rothballer, A. B. 1962. Brainstem localization of a neurohypophysial activating system in the cat. *Fed. Proc.* 21:353.

Kolff, W. J., and Page, I. H. 1954. Blood pressure reducing function of the kidney: reduction of renoprival hypertension by kidney perfusion. *Am. J. Physiol.* 178:75.

———, ———, and Corcoran, A. C. 1954. Pathogenesis of renoprival cardiovascular disease in dogs. *Am. J. Physiol.* 178:237.

Korner, P. I. 1971. Integrative neural cardiovascular control. *Physiol. Rev.* 51:312.

Koster, M. 1970. Patterns of hypertension. *Bibl. Psychiatr.* 144:1.

Kroneberg, G., and Shümann, H. J. 1959. Über die Bedeutung der Innervation für die Adrenalin-synthese in Nebennierenmark. *Experientia* 15:234.

Kubicek, W. G., Kottke, F. J., Laker, D. J., and Visscher, M. B. 1953. Adaptation in the pressor receptor reflex mechanisms in experimental neurogenic hypertension. *Am. J. Physiol.* 175:380.

Kuchel, O., Fishman, L. M., Liddle, G. W., and Michelakis, A. 1967. Effect of diazoxide on plasma renin activity in hypertensive patients. *Ann. Intern. Med.* 67:791.

Kurland, G. S., and Freedberg, A. S. 1951. The potentiating effect of ACTH and of cortisone on pressor response to intravenous infusion of L-norepinephrine. *Proc. Soc. Exp. Biol. Med.* 78:28.

Lacey, J. I. 1950. Individual differences in somatic response patterns. *J. Comp. Physiol. Psychol.* 43:338.

———— and Lacey, B. E. 1958. Verification and extension of the principle of autonomic response sterotypy. *Am. J. Psychol.* 71:50.

———— and Smith, R. L. 1954. Conditioning and generalization of unconscious anxiety. *Science* 120:1045.

———— and Van Lehn, R. 1952. Differential emphasis in somatic response to stress. An experimental study. *Psychosom. Med.* 14:71.

————, Bateman, D. E., and Van Lehn, R. 1953. Autonomic response specificity. An experimental study. *Psychosom. Med.* 15:8.

Lagerspetz, K. Y. H., Tirri, R., and Lagerspetz, K. M. J. 1967. Neurochemical and endocrinological studies of mice selectively bred for aggressiveness. *Rep. Inst. Psychol.* (Turku) 29:1.

Laidlaw, J. C., Yendt, E. R., and Gornall, A. G. 1963. Hypertension caused by renal artery occlusion simulating primary aldosteronism. *Metabolism* 9:612.

Lamprecht, F., Williams, R. B., and Kopin, I. J. 1973. Serum dopamine-beta-hydroxylase during development of immobilization-induced hypertension. *Endocrinology* 92:953.

————, Eichelman, B. S., Williams, R. B., Wooten, G. F., and Kopin, I. J. 1974. Serum dopamine-beta-hydroxylase (DBH) activity and blood pressure response of rat strains to shock-induced fighting. *Psychosom. Med.* 36:298.

Landau, W. M. 1953. Autonomic responses mediated via the corticospinal tract. *J. Neurophysiol.* 16:299.

Landgren, S. 1952. On the excitation mechanism of the carotid baroreceptors. *Acta Physiol. Scand.* 26:1.

Langford, H. G., Watson, R. L., and Douglas, B. H. 1968. Factors affecting blood pressure in population groups. *Trans. Assoc. Am. Physicians* 81:135.

Lapin, B. A. 1965. Response of the cardiovascular system of monkeys to stress. *Acta Cardiol.* (Brux.) 11:276.

Laragh, J. H. 1960. The role of aldosterone in man: evidence for regulation of electrolyte balance and arterial pressure by a renal-adrenal system which may be involved in malignant hypertension. *J.A.M.A.* 174:293.

———— 1961. Oversecretion of aldosterone in man and its relation to hypertensive vascular disease: Factors which control secretion of the hormone. In *Hypertension—Recent Advances: The Second Hahnemann Symposium on Hypertensive Disease,* edited by A. N. Brest and J. H. Moyer. Philadelphia: Lea & Febiger.

———— and Stoerk, H. C. 1957. A study of the mechanism of secretion of the sodium-retaining hormone (aldosterone). *J. Clin. Invest.* 36:383.

————, Angers, M., Kelly, W. G., and Lieberman, S. 1960. Hypotensive agents and pressor substances. The effect of epinephrine, norepinephrine, angiotensin II and others on the secretory rate of aldosterone in man. *J.A.M.A.* 174:234.

———, Sealey, J. E., and Sommers, S. C. 1966. Patterns of adrenal secretion and urinary excretion of aldosterone on plasma renin activity in normal and hypertensive subjects. *Circ. Res.* 18–19(Suppl. I):158.

———, ———, and Brunner, H. R. 1972. The control of aldosterone secretion in normal and hypertensive man: abnormal renin-aldosterone patterns in low renin hypertension. *Am. J. Med.* 53:549.

Laramore, D. C., and Grollman, A. 1950. Water and electrolyte content of tissues in normal and hypertensive rats. *Am. J. Physiol.* 161:278.

Laverty, R., and Smirk, F. H. 1961. Observations on the pathogenesis of spontaneous inherited hypertension and constricted renal-artery hypertension. *Circ. Res.* 9:455.

Leaf, R. C., Lerner, L., and Horovitz, Z. P. 1969. The role of the amygdala in the pharmacological and endocrinological manipulation of aggression. In *The Biology of Aggressive Behavior*, edited by S. Garattini and E. B. Sigg. Amsterdam: Excerpta Medica.

Ledingham, J. G. G., Bull, M. B., and Laragh, J. H. 1967. The meaning of aldosteronism in hypertensive disease. *Circ. Res.* 21 (Suppl. II):177.

Ledingham, J. M. 1971. Mechanisms in renal hypertension. *Proc. Roy. Soc. Med.* 64:409.

Ledsome, J. R., Linden, R. J., and O'Connor, W. J. 1961. The mechanisms by which distension of the left atrium produces diuresis in anesthetized dogs. *J. Physiol.* (Lond.) 159:87.

Lee, J. B., Gougoutos, J. Z., Takman, B. H., Daniels, E. G., Grostic, M. F., Pike, J. E., Hinman, J. W., and Muirhead, E. E. 1966. Vasodepressor and antihypertensive prostaglandins of PGE type with emphasis on the identification of medullin as PGE_2. *J. Clin. Invest.* 45:1036.

Lefer, A. M. 1973. Blood-borne humoral factors in the pathophysiology of circulatory shock. *Circ. Res.* 32:129.

Lehr, D., Goldman, H. W., and Casner, P. 1973. Renin-angiotensin role in thirst: paradoxical enhancement of drinking by angiotensin converting inhibitor. *Science* 182:1031.

Lenel, R., Katz, L. N., and Rodbard, S. 1948. Arterial hypertension in the chicken. *Am. J. Physiol.* 152:557.

Levy, R. L., White, P. D., Stroud, W. D., and Hillman, C. C. 1945. Transient hypertension: The relative prognostic importance of various systolic and diastolic levels. *J.A.M.A.* 128:1059.

Lew, E. A. 1967. Blood pressure and mortality—Life insurance experience. In *The Epidemiology of Hypertension: Proceedings of an Internatioal Symposium,* edited by J. Stamler, R. Stamler, and T. N. Pullman. New York: Grune & Stratton.

Lewinsohn, P. M. 1956. Personality correlates of duodenal ulcer and other psychosomatic reactions. *J. Clin. Psychol.* 12:296.

Lewis, G. P., and Piper, P. J. 1975. Inhibition of release of prostaglandins as an explanation of some of the actions of anti-inflammatory corticosteroids. *Nature* 254:308.

Lewis, P. J., Reid, J. L., Chalmers, J. P., and Dollery, C. T. 1973. Importance of central catecholaminergic neurons in the development of renal hypertension. *Clin. Sci. Mol. Med.* 45:115S.

Lindgren, P. 1955. The mesencephalon and the vasomotor system. *Acta Physiol. Scand.* 35 (Suppl.):121.

——— and Uvnäs, B. 1954. Photo-electric recording of the venous and arterial blood flow. *Acta Physiol. Scand.* 32:259.

Loewenstein, F. W. 1961. Blood pressure in relation to age and sex in the tropics and subtropics. A review of the literature and an investigation in two tribes of Brazil Indians. *Lancet* i:389.

Löfving, B. 1961. Cardiovascular adjustments induced from the rostral cingulate gyrus with special reference to sympatho-inhibitory mechanisms. *Acta Physiol. Scand.* 53 (Suppl. 184):1.

Louis, W. J. Spector, S., Tabei, R., and Sjoerdsma, A. 1968. Noradrenaline in the heart of the spontaneously hypertensive rats. *Lancet* i:1013.

———, Tabei, R., and Spector, S. 1971. Effects of sodium intake on inherited hypertension in the rat. *Lancet* ii:1283

Lovell, R. R. H. 1967. Race and blood pressure with special reference to Oceania. In *The Epidemiology of Essential Hypertension*, edited by J. Stamler, R. Stamler, and T. N. Pullman. New York: Grune & Stratton.

Lowenstein, J., Beranbaum, E. R., Chasis, H., and Baldwin, D. S. 1970. Intrarenal pressure and exaggerated natriuresis in essential hypertension. *Clin. Sci. Mol. Med.* 38:359.

Luetscher, J. A., Jr., and Axelrad, B. J. 1954. Increased aldosterone output during sodium deprivation in normal men. *Proc. Soc. Exp. Biol. Med.* 87:650.

———, Weinberger, M. H., Dowdy, A. J., Nokes, G. W., Balikian, H., Brodie, A., and Willoughby, S. 1969. Effects of sodium loading, sodium depletion and posture on plasma aldosterone concentration and renin activity in hypertensive patients. *J. Clin. Endocrinol.* 29:1310.

———, Boyers, D. G., Cuthbertson, J. G., and McMahon, D. F. 1973. A model of the human circulation. *Circ. Res.* 32, Suppl. I:I–84.

Lund, A. 1943. *Cortex Cerebris Betydning for Extremiteternes Vasomotoric.* Copenhagen: Munksgaard.

Lund-Johansen, P. 1967. Hemodynamics in early essential hypertension. *Acta Med. Scand.* Suppl. 482, 1.

Maas, J. W. 1962. Neurochemical differences between two strains of mice. *Science* 137:621.

McConnell, S. D., and Henkin, R. L. 1973. Increased preference for Na^+ and K^+ salts in spontaneously hypertensive (SH) rats. *Proc. Soc. Exp. Biol. Med.* 143:185.

McCubbin, J. W. 1958. Carotid sinus participation in experimental renal hypertension. *Circulation* 17:791.

——— and Page, I. H. 1958. Do ganglion-blocking agents and reserpine affect central vasomotor activity? *Circ. Res.* 6:816.

———, Green, J. H., and Page, I. H. 1956. Baroreceptor function in chronic renal hypertension. *Circ. Res.* 4:205.

McCubbin, J. W. 1967. Interrelationships between the sympathetic nervous system and the renin-angiotensin system. In *Baroreceptors and Hypertension*, edited by P. Kezdi. New York: Pergamon.

McDonald, R. K., Wagner, E. N., Jr., and Weise, V. K. 1957. Relationship between endogenous antidiuretic hormone activity and ACTH release in man. *Proc. Soc. Exp. Biol. Med.* 96:652.

McDonough, J., and Wilhelmj, C. M. 1954. The effect of excess salt intake on human blood pressure. *Am. J. Dig. Dis.* 21:180.

McGinn, N. F., Harburg, E., Julius, S., and MacLeod, J. M. 1964. Psychological correlates of blood pressure. *Psych. Bull.* 61:209.

McKegney, F. P., and Williams, R. B., Jr. 1967. Psychological aspects of hypertension: II. The differential influence of interview variables on blood pressure. *Am. J. Psychiatry* 123:1539.

McKenzie, J. K., and Phelan, E. L. 1969. Plasma and renin in the New Zealand strain of genetic hypertensive and random-bred control rats. *Proc. Univ. Otago Med. Sch.* 47:23.

MacKenzie, L. F., and Shepherd, P. 1937. The significance of past hypertension in applicants later presenting normal average blood pressures. *Proc. Med. Sect. Life Insur. Assoc.* 24:157.

McKusick, V. 1960. Genetics and the nature of essential hypertension. *Circulation* 22:857.

McQueen, J. D., Brown, K. M., and Walker, A. E. 1954. Role of the brainstem in blood pressure regulation in the dog. *Neurology* 4:1.

McSmythe, C., Nickel, J. F., and Bradley, S. E. 1952. The effect of epinephrine (USP), 1-epinephrine, and 1-norepinephrine on glomerular filtration rate, renal plasma flow, and the urinary excretion of sodium, potassium, and water in normal man. *J. Clin. Invest.* 31:499.

Maddocks, I. 1961. The influence of standard of living on blood pressure in Fiji. *Circulation* 24:1220.

Makarychev, A. I., and Kuritsa, A. I. 1951. Experimental hypertension of cortical origin. *Zh. Vyssh. Nerv. Deiat.* 1:199.

Malmo, R. B., and Shagass, C. 1952. Studies of blood pressure in psychiatric patients under stress. *Psychosom. Med.* 14:82.

Mason, J. W. 1968. The scope of psychoendocrine research. *Psychosom. Med.* Part 2, 30:565.

Masson, G. M. C., Mikasa, A., and Yasuda, H. 1962. Experimental vascular disease elicited by aldosterone and renin. *Endocrinology* 71:505.

Matarazzo, G. 1954. An experimental study of aggression in the hypertensive patient. *J. Pers.* 22:423.

Mathers, J. A. L., Osborne, R. H., and DeGeorge, F. V. 1961. Studies of blood pressure, heart rate, and the electrocardiogram in adult twins. *Am. Heart J.* 63:634.

Maynert, E. W., and Levi, R. 1964. Stress-induced release of brain norepinephrine and its inhibition by drugs. *J. Pharmacol. Exp. Ther.* 143:90.

Meehan, J. P. 1960. Central nervous control of the renal circulation. *Am. Heart J.* 6:318.

Mellander, S. 1960. Comparative studies on the adrenergic neuro-hormonal control of resistance and capacitance blood vessels in the cat. *Acta Physiol. Scand.* 176 Suppl.:1.

Mendlowitz, M. 1967. Vascular reactivity in essential and renal hypertension in man. *Am. Heart J.* 73:121.

———— and Naftchi, N. 1958. Work of digital vasoconstriction produced by infused norepinephrine in primary hypertension. *J. Appl. Physiol.* 13:247.

————, Gitlow, S., and Naftchi, N. 1958. Work of digital vasoconstriction produced by infused norepinephrine in Cushing's syndrome. *J. Appl. Physiol.* 13:252.

————, ————, and ———— 1959. The cause of essential hypertension. *Perspect. Biol. Med.* 2:354.

————, Naftchi, N., Weinreb, H. L., and Gitlow, S. E. 1961. Effect of prednisone on digital vascular reactivity in normotensive and hypertensive subjects. *J. Appl. Physiol.* 16:89.

Meneely, G. R., Tucker, R. G., Darby, W. J., and Auerbach, S. H. 1953. Chronic sodium chloride toxicity in the albino rat. II. Occurrence of hypertension and of a syndrome of edema and renal failure. *J. Exp. Med.* 98:71.

————, ————, ————, Ball, C. O. T., Kory, R. C., and Auerbach, S. H. 1954. Electrocardiographic changes, disturbed lipid metabolism and decreased survival rates observed in rats chronically eating increased sodium chloride. *Am. J. Med.* 16:599.

Merrill, J. P., Murray, J. E., Harrison, J. H., and Guild, W. R. 1956. Successful homotransplantation of the human kidney between identical twins. *J.A.M.A.* 160:277.

————, Giordano, C., and Heetderks, D. R. 1961. The role of the kidney in human hypertension. I. Failure of hypertension to develop in the renoprival subject. *Am. J. Med.* 31:931.

Mess, B. 1967. Endocrine and neurochemical aspects of pineal function. *Int. Rev. Neurobiol.* 11:171.

Meyer, P. H. (Discussant). 1967. The meaning of aldosteronism in hypertensive disease. *Circ. Res.* 21 (Suppl. II):186.

Miall, W. E., and Oldham, P. D. 1958. Factors influencing arterial blood pressure in the general population. *Clin. Sci.* 17:409.

————, Kass, E. H., Ling, J., and Stuart, K. L. 1962. Factors influencing arterial pressure in the general population in Jamaica. *Br. Med. J.* 2:497.

————, Heneage, P., Khosla, T., Lovell, H. G., and Moore, F. 1967. Factors influencing the degree of resemblance in arterial pressure of close relatives. *Clin. Sci.* 33:271.

Miasnikov, A. L. 1954. *Hypertensive Disease*. Moscow: Medgiz.

———— 1962. Significance of disturbances of higher nervous activity in the pathogenesis of hypertensive disease. In *Symposium on the Pathogenesis of Essential Hypertension*, edited by J. H. Cort, V. Fencl, Z. Hejl, and J. Jirka. New York: Pergamon.

Miles, B. E., and De Wardener, H. E. 1953. Effect of emotion on renal function in normotensive and hypertensive women. *Lancet* ii:539.

Miller, E. D., Jr., Samuels, A. I., Haber, E., and Barger, A. C. 1972. Inhibition of angiotensin conversion in experimental renovascular hypertension. *Science* 177:1108.

Miller, M. L. 1939. Blood pressure and inhibited aggression in psychotics. *Psychosom. Med.* 1:162.

Miller, N. E. 1969. Learning of visceral and glandular responses. *Science* 163:434.

Mills, E., and Wang, S. C. 1963. Localization of ascending pathways in the rostral brainstem of the dog for ADH liberation. *Fed. Proc.* 22:572.

Mills, L. C., Moyer, J. H., and Skelton, J. M. 1953. The effect of norepinephrine and epinephrine on renal hemodynamics. *Am. J. Med. Sci.* 226:653.

Miminoshvili, D. I. 1960. Experimental neurosis in monkeys. In *Theoretical and Practical Problems of Medicine in Biology in Experiments on Monkeys*, edited by I. A. Utkin. New York: Pergamon.

Mirsky, I. A., Stein, M., and Paulisch, G. 1954. The secretion of an antidiuretic substance into the circulation of rats exposed to noxious stimuli. *Endocrinology* 54:491.

Mogil, R. A., Irskovitz, H., Russell, J. H., and Murphy, J. J. 1969. Renal innervation and renin activity in salt metabolism and hypertension. *Am. J. Physiol.* 216:693.

Monroe, R. R., Heath, R. G., Head, R. G., Stone, R. L., and Ritter, K. A. 1961. A comparison of hypertensive and hypotensive schizophrenics. *Psychosom. Med.* 23:508.

Morgan, C. T., and Galambos, R. 1942. Production of audiogenic seizures by tones of low frequency. *Am. J. Psychol.* 55:555.

Morris, R. E., Jr., Ranson, P. A., and Howard, J. E. 1962. Studies on the relationship of angiotensin to hypertension of renal origin. *J. Clin. Invest.* 41:1386.

Moruzzi, G. 1940. Paleocerebellar inhibition of vasomotor and respiratory carotid sinus reflexes. *J. Neurophysiol.* 3:20.

———— 1950. *Problems in Cerebellar Physiology*. Springfield, Ill.: Charles C Thomas.

Moschowitz, E. 1919. Hypertension: its significance, relation to arteriosclerosis and nephritis, and etiology. *Am. J. Med. Sci.* 158:668.

Moses, L., Daniels, G. E., and Nickerson, J. L. 1956. Psychogenic factors in essential hypertension: Methodology and preliminary report. *Psychosom. Med.* 18:471.

Muirhead, E. E., Brooks, B., Kosinski, M., Daniels, E. E., and Hinman, J. W. 1966. Renomedullary antihypertensive principle in renal hypertension. *J. Lab. Clin. Med.* 67:778.

————, Leach, B. E., Brown, G. B., Daniels, E. G., and Hinman, J. W. 1967. Antihypertensive effect of prostaglandin E2 (PGE2) in renovascular hypertension. *J. Lab. Clin. Med.* 70:986.

————, Brown, G. B., Germain, G. S., and Leach, B. E. 1970. The renal medulla as an antihypertensive organ. *J. Lab. Clin. Med.* 76:641.

Muller, A. F., Manning, E. L., and Riondel, A. M. 1958. Influence of position and activity on the secretion of aldosterone. *Lancet* i:711.

Mulrow, P. J., Ganong, W. F., Cera, G., and Kulgian, A. 1962. The nature of the aldosterone-stimulating factor in dog kidneys. *J. Clin. Invest.* 41:505.

Murray, J. E., Merrill, J. P., and Harrison, J. H. 1958. Kidney transplantation between seven pairs of identical twins. *Ann. Surg.* 148:343.

Nagareda, C. S., and Gaunt, R. 1951. Functional relationship between the adrenal cortex and posterior pituitary. *Endocrinology* 48:560.

Nakamura, K., Gerold, M., and Thoenen, H. 1971. Experimental hypertension of the rat: Reciprocal changes of norepinephrine turnover in heart and brainstem. *Naunyn-Schmiedebergs Arch. Pharmacol.* 268:125.

———, ———, and ———. 1971. Genetically hypertensive rats: Relationship between the development of hypertension and the changes in norepinephrine turnover of peripheral and central adrenergic neurons. *Naunyn-Schmiedebergs Arch. Pharmacol.* 271:157.

Napalkov, A. V., and Karas, I. 1957. Abolishment of pathologic conditioned associations in experimental hypertension. *Zh. Vysshei Nerv. Deiat.* 7:402.

Neiberg, N. A. 1957. The effects of induced stress on the management of hostility in essential hypertension. *Dissert. Abstr.* 17:1597.

Nestel, P. J. 1969. Blood pressure and catecholamine excretion after mental stress in labile hypertension. *Lancet* i:692.

Neumayr, R. J., Hare, B. D., and Franz, D. N. 1974. Evidence for bulbospinal control of sympathetic preganglionic neurons by monoaminergic pathways. *Life Sci.* 14:793.

Newton, M. A., and Laragh, J. H. 1968a. Effect of corticotropin on aldosterone excretion and plasma renin in normal subjects, in essental hypertension and in primary aldosteronism. *J. Clin. Endocrinol. Metab.* 28:1006.

——— and ——— 1968b. Effects of glucocorticoid administration on aldosterone excretion and plasma renin in normal subjects, in essential hypertension and in primary aldosteronism. *J. Clin. Endocrinol. Metab.* 28:1014.

Nicotero, J. A., Beamer, V., Moutsos, S. E., and Shapiro, A. P. 1968. Effects of propranolol on the pressor response to noxious stimuli in hypertensive patients. *Am. J. Cardiol.* 22:657.

Norberg, K.-A. 1967. Transmitter histochemistry of the sympathetic adrenergic nervous system. *Brain Res.* 5:125.

O'Connor, W. J., and Verney, E. B. 1945. The effect of increased activity of the sympathetic system in the inhibition of water diuresis by emotional stress. *Q. J. Exp. Physiol.* 33:77.

O'Hare, J. P. 1920. Vascular reactions in vascular hypertension. *Am. J. Med. Sci.* 159:371.

———, Walker, W. G., and Vickers, M. C. 1924. Heredity and hypertension. *J.A.M.A.* 83:27.

Okamoto, K. 1969. Spontaneous hypertension in rats. *Int. Rev. Exp. Pathol.* 7:227.

——— and Aoki, K. 1963. Development of a strain of spontaneously hypertensive rats. *Jpn. Circ. J.* 27:282.

Oliver, J. T., Birmingham, M. K., Bartova, A., Li, M. P., and Chan, T. H. 1973. Hypertensive action of 18-hydroxydeoxycorticosterone. *Science* 182:1249.

Orbison, J. L., Christian, C. L., and Peters, E. 1952. Studies on experimental hypertension and cardiovascular disease. *Arch. Pathol.* 54:185.

Orlov, V. V. 1959. On mechanics of influence of cerebral cortex on reaction of peripheral vessels. *Zh. Vysshei Nerv. Deiat.* 9:712.

Ostfeld, A. M. 1973. Editorial: What's the payoff in hypertension research? *Psychosom. Med.* 35:1.

——— and Lebovitz, B. Z. 1959. Personality factors and pressor mechanisms in renal and essential hypertension. *Arch. Intern. Med.* 104:497.

——— and ——— 1960. Blood pressure lability: a correlative study. *J. Chronic Dis.* 12:428.

——— and Paul, O. 1963. The inheritance of hypertension. *Lancet* i:575.

——— and Shekelle, R. B. 1967. Psychological variables and blood pressure. In *The Epidemiology of Essential Hypertension*, edited by J. Stamler, R. Stamler, and T. N. Pullman. New York: Grune & Stratton.

Padmavati, S., and Gupta, S. 1959. Blood pressure studies in rural and urban groups in Delhi. *Circulation* 19:395.

Page, I. H. 1935. Relationship of extrinsic venal nerves to origin of experimental hypertension. *Am. J. Physiol.* 112:166.

——— 1960. The mosaic theory of hypertension. In *Essential Hypertension*, edited by K. D. Bock and P. T. Cottier. Berlin: Springer.

——— and McCubbin, J. W. 1951. The pattern of vascular reactivity in experimental hypertension of varied origin. *Circulation* 4:70.

111

———— and ———— 1965. The physiology of hypertension. In *Handbook of Physiology*, Sect. 2: Circulation. American Physiological Society.

Palmer, R. S. 1930. The significance of essential hypertension in young male adults. *J.A.M.A.* 94:694.

———— 1950. Psyche and blood pressure. *J.A.M.A.* 144:295.

Papez, J. W. 1926. Reticulo-spinal tracts in the cat. Marchi method. *J. Comp. Neurol.* 41:365.

Passo, S. S., Assaykeen, T. A., Orsuka, K., Wise, B. L., Goldfien, A., and Ganong, W. F. 1971. Effect of stimulation of the medulla oblongata on renin secretion in dogs. *Neuroendocrinology* 7:1.

Patterson, G. C., Shepard, J. T., and Whelan, R. F. 1957. Resistance to flow in the upper and lower limb vessels in patients with coarctation of the aorta. *Clin. Sci.* 16:627.

Paulsen, E. C., and Hess, S. M. 1963. The rate of synthesis of catecholamines following depletion in guinea pig brain and heart. *J. Neurochem.* 10:453.

Peart, W. S. 1959. Hypertension and the kidney. I. Clinical, pathological, and functional disorders, especially in man. II. Experimental basis of renal hypertension. *Br. Med. J.* ii:1353; 1421.

Perera, G. W. 1955. Hypertensive vascular disease: description and natural history. *J. Chronic Dis.* 1:33.

————, Clark, E. G., Gearing. F. R., and Schweitzer, M. D. 1961. The family of hypertensive man. *Am. J. Med. Sci.* 241:18.

Perlmutt, J. H. 1963. Reflex diuresis after occlusion of common carotid arteries in hydrated dogs. *Am. J. Physiol.* 204:197.

Peterson, L. H. 1961. Hemodynamic alterations in essential hypertension. In *Hypertension-Recent Advances. The Second Hahnemann Symposium on Hypertensive Disease*, edited by A. N. Brest and J. H. Moyer. Philadelphia: Lea & Febiger.

———— 1963. Systems behavior, feed-back loops and high blood pressure research. *Circ. Res.* 12:585.

Petyelina, V. V. 1952. Conditional reflexive influences on blood vessels and respiration during strenuous mental activity. *Fiziol. Zh. SSSR* 38:566.

Pfeffer, M. A., and Frohlich, E. D. 1973. Hemodynamic and myocardial function in young and old normotensive and spontaneously hypertensive rats. *Circ. Res.* 32(Suppl. I):28.

Pfeiffer, J. B., Jr., and Wolff, H. G. 1950. Studies in renal circulation during periods of life stress and accompanying emotional reactions in subjects with and without essential hypertension: Observations on the role of neural activity in the regulation of renal blood flow. *Res. Publ. Assoc. Res. Nerv. Ment. Dis.* 29:929.

Pickering, G. W. 1945. Role of kidney in acute and chronic hypertension following renal artery constriction in rabbit. *Clin. Sci.* 5:229.

———— 1955. *High Blood Pressure*. London: Churchill.

———— 1961. *The Nature of Essential Hypertension*. New York: Grune & Stratton.

———— 1967. The inheritance of arterial pressure. In *The Epidemiology of Hypertension*, edited by J. Stamler, R. Stamler, and T. N. Pullman. New York: Grune & Stratton.

Pickford, M. 1952. Antidiuretic substances. *Pharmacol. Rev.* 4:255.

Pilowsky, I., Spalding, D., Shaw, J., and Korner, P. I. 1973. Hypertension and personality. *Psychosom. Med.* 35:50.

Pitts, R. F., and Bronk, D. W. 1941/1942. Excitability cycle of the hypothalamus-sympathetic neurone system. *Am. J. Physiol.* 135:504.

————, Larrabee, M. G., and Bronk, D. W. 1941. An analysis of hypothalamic cardiovascular control. *Am. J. Physiol.* 134:359.

Platt, R. 1947. Heredity in hypertension. *Q. J. Med.* 16:111.

———— 1959. The nature of essential hypertension. *Lancet* ii:55.

———— 1963. Heredity in hypertension. *Lancet* i:899.

———— 1967. The influence of heredity. In *The Epidemiology of Essential Hypertension*, edited by J. Stamler, R. Stamler, and T. N. Pullman. New York: Grune & Stratton.

Pool, J. L., and Ransohoff, J. 1949. Autonomic effects on stimulating rostral portion of cingulate gyri in man. *J. Neurophysiol.* 12:385.

Ramey, E. R., Goldstein, M. S., and Levine, R. 1951. Action of nor-epinephrine and adrenal cortical steroids on blood pressure and work performance of adrenalectomized dogs. *Am. J. Physiol.* 165:450.

Rankin, E. M., and Pappenheimer, J. R. 1957. Wasserdurchlässigkeit und Permeabilitet der Kapillarwande. *Ergeb. Physiol.* 49:59.

Ranson, S. W., and Billingsley, P. R. 1916. Vasomotor reactions from stimulation of the floor of the fourth ventricle. *Am. J. Physiol.* 41:85.

Rapp, J. P., and Dahl, L. K. 1971. Adrenal steroidogenesis in rats bred for susceptibility and resistance to the hypertensive effect of salt. *Endocrinology* 88:52.

———— and ———— 1972. Possible role of 18-hydroxycorticosterone in hypertension. *Nature* 237:338.

————, Knudsen, K. D., Iwai, J., and Dahl, L. K. 1973. Genetic control of blood pressure and corticosteroid production in rats. *Circ. Res.* 32(Suppl. I):139.

Redleaf, P., and Tobian, L. 1958a. The question of vascular hyperresponsiveness in hypertension. *Circ. Res.* 6:185.

———— and ———— 1958b. Sodium restriction and reserpine administration in experimental renal hypertension. A correlation of arterial blood pressure responses with the ionic composition of the arterial wall. *Circ. Res.* 6:343.

Redmond, D. P., Gaylor, M. S., McDonald, R. H., Jr., and Shapiro, A. P. 1974. Blood pressure and heart-rate response to verbal instruction and relaxation in hypertension. *Psychosom. Med.* 36:285.

Reed, R. K., Sapirstein, L. A., Southard, F. D., Jr., and Ogden, E. 1944. The effects of nembutal and yohimbine on chronic renal hypertension in the rat. *Am. J. Physiol.* 141:707.

Reese, W. G., and Dykman, R. A. 1960. Conditional cardiovascular reflexes in dogs and men. *Physiol. Rev.* 40(Suppl. 4):250.

Reiser, M. F. 1970. Theoretical considerations of the role of psychological factors in pathogenesis and etiology of essential hypertension. *Bibl. Psychiatr.* 144:117.

————, Brust, A. A., Shapiro, A. P., Baker, H. M., Ranschoff, W., and Ferris, E. B. 1950. Life situations, emotions and the course of patients with arterial hypertension. *Res. Publ. Assoc. Res. Nerv. Ment. Dis.* 29:870.

————, ————, and Ferris, E. B. 1951a. Life situations, emotions and the course of patients with arterial hypertension. *Psychosom. Med.* 13:133.

————, Rosenbaum, M., and Ferris, E. B. 1951b. Psychologic mechanisms in malignant hypertension. *Psychosom. Med.* 13:147.

Remington, R. D., Lambarth, B., Moser, M., and Hoobler, S. W., 1960. Circulatory reactions of normotensive and hypertensive subjects and of the children of normal and hypertensive parents. *Am. Heart J.* 59:58.

Robinson, J. O. 1962. A study of neuroticism and casual arterial blood pressure. *Br. J. Clin. Psychol.* 2:56.

———— 1964. A possible effect of selection on the test scores of a group of hypertensives. *J. Psychosom. Res.* 8:239.

———— 1969. Symptoms and the discovery of high blood pressure. *J. Psychosom. Res.* 13:157.

Robinson, S. C., and Brucer, M. 1939. Range of normal blood pressure, statistical study of 11,383 persons. *Arch. Intern. Med.* 6:409.

Rochlin, D. B., Shohl, T. E., and Cary, A. L. 1959. A comparison of (Cr 51) blood volumes in hypertensive and normal patients. *Fed. Proc.* 18:129.

Rosenman, R. H. 1969. The possible general causes of coronary artery disease. In *Pathogenesis of Coronary Artery Disease*, edited by M. Friedman. New York: McGraw-Hill.

——— and Friedman, M. 1963. Behavior patterns, blood lipids, and coronary heart disease. *J.A.M.A.* 184:934.

———, ———, Straus, R., Wurm, M., Kositechek, R., Hahn, W., and Werthessen, N. T. 1964. A predictive study of coronary heart disease. *J.A.M.A.* 189:15.

———, ———, ———, ———, Jenkins, D., and Messinger, H. 1966. Coronary heart disease in the Western Collaborative Group Study. *J.A.M.A.* 195:86.

Rosenthal, J., Paddock, J., and Hollander, W. 1973. Identification of a new vasodepressor factor (VDF) in arterial tissue and plasma of dogs and humans. *Circ. Res.* 32(Suppl. I):I–169.

Ross, E. J. 1960. Modification of the effects of aldosterone on electrolyte excretion in man by simultaneous administration of corticosterone and hydrocortisone. Relevance to Conn's syndrome. *J. Clin. Endocrinol.* 20:229.

Rossi, G. F., and Brodal, A. 1956. Corticofugal fibres to brain-stem reticular formation; experimental study in cat. *J. Anat.* (Lond.) 90:42.

Rothballer, A. 1966. Pathways of secretion and regulation of posterior pituitary factors. *Res. Publ. Assoc. Res. Nerv. Ment. Dis.* 43:86.

Rothlin, E., Emmenger, H., and Cerletti, A. 1953. Experiments to próduce essential hypertension in rats. *Helv. Physiol. Pharmacol. Acta* 11:C25.

———, Cerletti, A., and Emmenger, H. 1956. Experimental psychoneurogenic hypertension and its treatment with hydrogenated ergotalkaloids (Hydrergine). *Acta Med. Scand.* 312(Suppl.):27.

Rovner, D. R., Conn, J. W., Knopf, R. F., Cohen, E. L., and Hsueh, M. T.-Y. 1965. Nature of renal escape from the sodium-retaining effects of aldosterone in primary aldosteronism and in normal subjects. *J. Clin. Endocrinol. Metab.* 25:53.

Rushmer, R. F. 1958. Heart adaptation to environment. Neural and humoral control of the heart. *Abstracts of the Symposium, World Congress of Cardiology.* Brussels.

Ruskin, A., Beard, O. W., and Schaffer, R. L. 1948. "Blast hypertension": Elevated arterial pressure in victims of the Texas City disaster. *Am. J. Med.* 4:228.

Russi, S., Blumenthal, H. T., and Gray, S. H. 1945. Small adenomas of the adrenal cortex in hypertension and diabetes. *Arch. Intern. Med.* 76:284.

Rydin, H., and Verney, E. B. 1938. The inhibition of water-diuresis by emotional stress and by muscular exercise. *Q. J. Exp. Physiol.* 27:343.

Ryvkin, I. A. 1960. The role of heredity in the etiology of hypertensive vascular disease. *Klin. Med.* (Moskva) 38:24.

Sachs, E., Jr., Brendler, S. J., and Fulton, J. F. 1949. The orbital gyri. *Brain* 72:227.

Saffran, M., Schally, A. V., and Benfey, B. G. 1955. Stimulation of the release of corticotropin from the adenohypophysis by a neurohypophysial factor. *Endocrinology* 57:439.

Sainsbury, P. 1960. Psychosomatic disorders and neurosis in out-patients attending a general hospital. *J. Psychosom. Res.* 4:261.

——— 1964. Neuroticism and hypertension in an out-patient population. *J. Psychosom. Res.* 8:235.

Sannerstedt, R. 1969. Hemodynamic findings at rest and during exercise in mild arterial hypertension. *Am. J. Med. Sci.* 258:70.

Sapira, J. D., Lipman, R. L., and Shapiro, A. P. 1966. Hyperresponsivity to angiotensin induced in rats by behavioral stimulation. *Proc. Soc. Exp. Biol. Med.* 123:52.

———, Scheib, E. T., Moriarty, R., and Shapiro, A. P. 1971. Differences in perception between hypertensive and normotensive populations. *Psychosom. Med.* 33:239.

Sapirstein, L. A. 1957. Sodium and water ratios in the pathogenesis of hypertension. *Proc. Coun. High Blood Press. Res.* 6:28.

———, Brandt, W. L., and Drury, D. R. 1950. Production of hypertension in rat by substituting hypertonic sodium chloride solutions for drinking water. *Proc. Soc. Exp. Biol. Med.* 73:82.

Saslow, G., Gressel, G. C., Shobe, F. O., Dubois, P. H., and Schroeder, H. A. 1950. Possible etiological relevance of personality factors in hypertension. *Psychosom. Med.* 12:292.

Saul, L. J. 1939. Hostility in cases of essential hypertension. *Psychosom. Med.* 1:153.

Schachter, J. 1957. Pain, fear and anger in hypertensives and normotensives: A psychophysiologic study. *Psychosom. Med.* 19:17.

Schechter, P. J., Horwitz, D., and Henkin, R. I. 1973. Sodium chloride preference in essential hypertension. *J.A.M.A.* 225:1311.

Schlager, G. 1966. Systolic blood pressure in eight inbred strains of mice. *Nature* 212:519.

Schmiterlow, C. G. 1948. Nature and occurrence of pressor and depressor substances in extracts from blood vessels. *Acta Physiol. Scand.* (Suppl.)56:1.

Schwartz, S. I., and Griffith, L. S. C. 1967. Reduction of hypertension by electrical stimulation of the carotid sinus nerve. In *Baroreceptors and Hypertension*, edited by P. Kezdi. New York: Pergamon.

Schweitzer, M. D., Gearing, F. R., and Perera, G. A. 1967. Family studies of primary hypertension: their contribution to the understanding of genetic factors. In *The Epidemiology of Essential Hypertension*, edited by J. Stamler, R. Stamler, and T. N. Pullman. New York: Grune & Stratton.

Scotch, N. A. 1961. Blood pressure measurements of urban Zulu adults. *Am. Heart J.* 61:173.

——— and Geiger, J. H. 1963. Epidemiology of essential hypertension: psychologic and sociocultural factors in etiology. *J. Chronic Dis.* 16:1183.

Scroop, G. C., and Lowe, R. D. 1968. Central pressor effect of angiotensin mediated by the parasympathetic nervous system. *Nature* 220:331.

Selye, H., Hall, C. E., and Rowley, E. M. 1943. Malignant hypertension produced by treatment with desoxycorticosterone acetate and sodium chloride. *Can. Med. Assoc. J.* 49:88.

Sen, S., Smeby, R. R., and Bumpus, F. M. 1972. Renin in rats with spontaneous hypertension. *Circ. Res.* 31:876.

Shamma, A. H., Goodard, J. W., and Sommers, S. C. 1958. A study of the adrenal states in hypertension. *J. Chron. Dis.* 8:587.

Shapiro, A. P. 1960a. Comparative studies of the blood pressure response to different noxious stimuli. *Psychosom. Med.* 22:320.

——— 1960b. Psychophysiologic mechanisms in hypertensive vascular disease. *Ann. Intern. Med.* 53:64.

——— 1963. Experimental pyelonephritis and hypertension. *Ann. Intern. Med.* 59:37.

——— 1973. Essential hypertension—Why idiopathic? *Am. J. Med.* 54:1.

——— and Grollman, A. 1953. A critical evaluation of the hypotensive action of hydrallazine, hexamethonium, tetraethylammonium and dibenzyline salts in human and experimental hypertension. *Circulation* 8:188.

——— and Horn, P. W. 1955. Blood pressure, plasma pepsinogen, and behavior in cats subjected to experimental production of anxiety. *J. Nerv. Ment. Dis.* 122:222.

——— and Melhado, J. 1957. Factors affecting development of hypertensive vascular disease after renal injury in rats. *Proc. Soc. Exp. Biol. Med.* 96:619.

——— and Teng, H. C. 1957. Technic of controlled drug assay illustrated by a comparative study of rauwolfia serpentina, phenobarbital and placebo in the hypertensive patient. *N. Engl. J. Med.* 256:970.

———, Rosenbaum, M., and Ferris, E. B. 1954. Comparison of blood pressure response to veriloid and to the doctor. *Psychosom. Med.* 16:478.

115

————, Perez-Stable, E., Scheib, E. T., Broń, K., Moutsos, S. E., Berg, G., Misage, J. R., Bahnson, H., Fisher, B., and Drapanas, T. 1969. Renal artery stenosis and hypertension: Observations on current status of therapy from a study of 115 patients. *Am. J. Med.* 47:175.

Shapiro, D., Tursky, B., Gershon, E., and Stern, M. 1969. Effects of feedback and reinforcement on the control of human systolic blood pressure. *Science* 163:588.

————, Schwartz, G. E., and Tursky, B. 1970. Control of diastolic blood pressure in man by feedback and reinforcement. *Psychophysiology* 8:262.

Share, L., and Levy, M. N. 1962. Cardiovascular receptors and blood titer of antidiuretic hormone. *Am. J. Physiol.* 203:425.

Shekelle, R. B., Ostfeld, A. M., Lebovitz, B. Z., and Paul, O. 1970. Personality traits and coronary heart disease: a re-examination of Ibrahim's hypothesis using longitudinal data. *J. Chronic. Dis.* 23:33.

Sheldon, S. H., and Ball, R. 1950. Physiological characteristics of the Y twins and their relation to hypertension. *Res. Publ. Assoc. Res. Nerv. Ment. Dis.* 29:962.

Short, D. 1966. Morphology of the intestinal arterioles in chronic human hypertension. *Br. Heart J.* 28:184.

Simonson, E., and Brožek, J. 1959. Russian research on arterial hypertension. *Ann. Intern. Med.* 50:129.

Simpson, F. O., and Gilchrist, A. R. 1958. Prognosis in untreated hypertensive vascular disease. *Scott. Med. J.* 3:1.

Sinaiko, A., and Mirkin, B. L. 1974. Ontogenesis of the renin-angiotensin system in spontaneously hypertensive and normal Wistar rats. *Circ. Res.* 34:693.

Sivertsson, R. 1970. The hemodynamic importance of structural vascular changes in essential hypertension. *Acta Physiol. Scand.* Suppl. 343, 1.

Skinner, S. L., McCubbin, J. W., and Page, I. H. 1963. Route of renin release. *Fed. Proc.* 22:181.

Smirk, F. A. 1957. *High Arterial Pressure*. Springfield, Ill.: Charles C Thomas.

Smirk, F. H., and Hall, W. H. 1958. Inherited hypertension in rats. *Nature* 182:727.

Smith, H. W. 1939/1940. Physiology of the renal circulation. *Harvey Lect.* 35:166.

Smith, K. 1954. Conditioning as an artifact. *Psychol. Rev.* 61:217.

Sokolow, M., and Harris, R. E. 1961. The natural history of hypertensive disease. In *Hypertension—Recent Advances: The Second Hahnemann Symposium on Hypertensive Disease,* edited by A. N. Brest and J. H. Moyer. Philadelphia: Lea & Febiger.

———— and Perloff, D. B. 1961. The prognosis of essential hypertension treated conservatively. *Circulation* 23:697.

————, Werdegar, D., Perloff, D. B., Cowan, R. M., and Brenenstuhl, H. 1970. Preliminary studies relating portably recorded blood pressures to daily life events in patients with essential hypertension. *Bibl. Psychiatr.* 144:164.

Speransky, I. I., Soulie, E. U., and Bitkova, S. I. 1959. Hereditary-familial data on patients with hypertension. *Ter. Arkh.* 31:7.

Stamler, J., Lindberg, N. A., Berkson, D. M., Schaffer, A., Miller, W., and Poindexter, A. 1958. Epidemiological analysis of hypertension and hypertensive disease in the labor force of a Chicago utility company. *Hypertension* 7:23.

————, Berkson, D. M., Lindberg, H. A., Miller, W. A., Stamler, R., and Collette, R. 1967a. Socioeconomic factors in the epidemiology of hypertensive disease. In *The Epidemiology of Hypertension,* edited by J. Stamler, R. Stamler, and T. N. Pullman. New York: Grune & Stratton.

————, Stamler, R., and Pullman, T. 1967b. *The Epidemiology of Essential Hypertension.* New York: Grune & Stratton.

Stewart, I. McD. G. 1953. Headache and hypertension. *Lancet* i:1261.

116

Stone, E. A. 1970. Swim-stress-induced inactivity: relation to brain norepinephrine and body temperature, and effects of d-amphetamine. *Psychosom. Med.* 32:51.

Storment, C. T. 1951. Personality and heart disease. *Psychosom. Med.* 13:304.

Stott, A. W., and Robinson, R. 1967. Urinary normetadrenaline excretion in essential hypertension. *Clin. Chim. Acta* 16:249.

Streeten, D. H. P., Schletter, F. E., Clift, G. V., Stevenson, C. T., and Dalakos, T. G. 1969. Studies of the renin-angiotensin-aldosterone system in patients with hypertension and in normal subjects. *Am. J. Med.* 46:844.

Strong, C. G., Boucher, R., Nowaczynski, W., and Genest, J. 1966. Renal vasodepressor lipid. *Mayo Clin. Proc.* 41:433.

Suda, I., Koizumi, K., and Brooks, C. McC. 1963. Study of unitary activity in the supraoptic nucleus of the hypothalamus. *Jpn. J. Physiol.* 13:374.

Sweet, C. S., and Brody, M. J. 1971. Arterial hypertension elicited by prolonged intravertebral infusion of angiotensin in the conscious dog. *Fed. Proc.* 30:432.

————, and ———— 1970. Central inhibition of reflex vasodilation by angiotensin and reduced renal pressure. *Am. J. Physiol.* 219:1751.

Syme, S. L., Hyman, M. M., and Enterline, P. E. 1964. Some social and cultural factors associated with the occurrence of coronary heart disease. *J. Chronic Dis.* 17:277.

Takahashi, E., Sasaki, N., Takeda, J., and Ito, H. 1957. Geographic distribution of cerebral hemorrhage and hypertension in Japan. *Hum. Biol.* 29:139.

Taquini, A. C., Jr., Blaquier, P., and Bohr, D. F. 1961. Neurogenic factors and angiotensin in the etiology of hypertension. *Am. J. Physiol.* 201:1173.

Thaler, M., Weiner, H., and Reiser, M. F. 1957. Exploration of the doctor-patient relationship through projective techniques. *Psychosom. Med.* 19:228.

Thoenen, H., Mueller, R. A., and Axelrod, J. 1969. Trans-synaptic induction of adrenal tyrosine hydroxylase. *J. Pharmacol. Exp.* 169:249.

Thomas, C. B. 1957. Characteristics of the individual as guideposts to the prevention of heart disease. *Ann. Intern. Med.* 47:389.

———— 1958. Familial and epidemiologic aspects of coronary disease and hypertension. *J. Chronic Dis.* 7:198.

———— 1961. Pathogenetic interrelations in hypertension and coronary artery disease. *Dis. Nerv. Syst.* 22(Suppl.):39.

———— 1964a. Psychophysiologic aspects of blood pressure regulation: A clinician's view. *J. Chronic Dis.* 17:599.

———— 1964b. Psychophysiological aspects of blood pressure regulation: the clinician's view. *Psychosom. Med.* 26:454.

———— 1967. The psychological dimensions of hypertension. In *The Epidemiology of Essential Hypertension,* edited by J. Stamler, R. Stamler, and T. N. Pullman. New York: Grune & Stratton.

———— and Cohen, B. H. 1955. The familial occurrence of hypertension and coronary artery disease, with observations concerning obesity and diabetes. *Ann. Intern. Med.* 42:90.

———— and Ross, D. C. 1963. A new approach to the Rorschach test as a research tool. *Bull. Johns Hopkins Hosp.* 112:312.

————, Ross, D. C., and Higinbotham. C. Q. 1964a. Precursors of hypertension and coronary disease among healthy medical students; discriminant function analysis. II. Using parental history as the criterion. *Bull. Johns Hopkins Hosp.* 115:245.

————, Ross, D. C., and Freed, E. S. 1964b. *An Index of Rorschach Responses: Studies on the Psychological Characteristics of Medical Students.* Baltimore: Johns Hopkins University Press.

Thomson, K. J. 1950. Some observations on the development and course of hypertensive vascular disease. *Proc. Sect. Am. Life Insur. Assoc.*

Tobian, L. 1950. Hypertension following bilateral nephrectomy. *J. Clin. Invest.* 29:849.

———— 1960. Interrelationship of electrolytes, juxtaglomerular cells and hypertension. *Physiol. Rev.* 40:280.

———— 1961. The relationship of sodium to hypertension (clinical observations). In *Hypertension—Recent Advances. The Second Hahnemann Symposium on Hypertensive Disease,* edited by A. N. Brest, and J. H. Moyer. Philadelphia: Lea & Febiger.

———— 1962. Relationship of the juxtaglomerular apparatus to renin and angiotensin. *Circulation* 25:189.

———— 1972. A viewpoint concerning the enigma of hypertension. *Am. J. Med.* 52:595.

———— 1974. Experimental models for the study of hypertension. *Hosp. Pract.* 9:99.

———— and Azar, S. 1971. Antihypertensive and other functions of the renal papilla. *Trans. Assoc. Am. Physicians* 84:281.

———— and Binion, J. T. 1952. Tissue cations and water in arterial hypertension. *Circulation* 5:754.

———— and Chesley, G. 1966. Calcium content of arteriolar walls in normotensive and hypertensive rats. *Proc. Soc. Exp. Biol. Med.* 121:340.

————, Janecek, J., Tomboulian, A., and Ferreira, D. 1961. Sodium and potassium in the walls of arterioles in experimental renal hypertension. *J. Clin. Invest.* 40:1922.

————, Schonning, S., and Seefeldt, C. 1964. The influence of arterial pressure on the antihypertensive action of a normal kidney, a biological servo mechanism. *Ann. Intern. Med.* 60:378.

————, Olson, R., and Chesley, G. 1969a. Water content of arteriolar wall in renovascular hypertension. *Am. J. Physiol.* 216:22.

————, Ishii, M., and Duke, M. 1969b. Relationship of cytoplasmic granules in renal papillary interstitial cells to "post-salt" hypertension. *J. Lab. Clin. Med.* 73:309.

Toh, C. C. 1960. Effects of temperature on the 5-hydroxytryptamine content of tissues. *J. Physiol.* (Lond.) 151:410.

Tomaszewski, W. 1937. Puls- und Atmungsfrequenz unter psychischer Beeinflussung. *Z. Kreislaufforsch.* 29:745.

Torgersen, S., and Kringlen, E. 1971. Blood pressure and personality. A study of the relationship between intrapair differences in systolic blood pressure and personality in monozygotic twins. *J. Psychosom. Res.* 15:183.

Tucker, W. I. 1949. Psychiatric factors in essential hypertension. *Dis. Nerv. Syst.* 10:273.

———— 1950. Psychiatric factors in essential hypertension. *N. Engl. J. Med.* 243:211.

Ulick, S., Laragh, J. H., and Lieberman, S. 1958. The isolation of a urinary metabolite of aldosterone and its use to measure the rate of secretion of aldosterone by the adrenal cortex of man. *Trans. Assoc. Am. Physicians* 71:225.

Ulrych, M., Frohlich, E. D., Dustan, H. P., and Page, I. H. 1968. Immediate hemodynamic effects of beta-adrenergic blockade with propranolol in normotensive and hypertensive man. *Circulation* 37:411.

Usami, S., Peric, B., and Chien, S. 1962. Release of antidiuretic hormone due to common carotid occlusion and its relation with vagus nerve. *Proc. Soc. Exp. Biol. Med.* 111:189.

Uvnäs, B. 1960. Central cardiovascular control: In *Handbook of Physiology,* Sect. 1: Neurophysiology, vol. 2, chapt. 44. American Physiological Society.

Vander, A. J., and Miller, R. 1964. Control of renin secretion in the dog. *Am. J. Physiol.* 207:537.

Van Der Valk, J. M. 1957. Blood pressure changes under emotional influences in patients with essential hypertension and control subjects. *J. Psychosom. Res.* 2:134.

Vandongen, R., Peart, W. S., and Boyd, G. W. 1973. Adrenergic stimulation of renin secretion in the isolated perfused rat kidney. *Circ. Res.* 32:290.

Vermeulen, A., and Van der Straeten, M. 1963. Adrenal cortical function in benign essential hypertension. *J. Clin. Endocrinol. Metab.* 23:574.

118

Verney, E. B. 1947. Croonian lecture: The antidiuretic hormone and the factors which determine its release. *Proc. R. Soc. Lond.* [Biol.] 135:25.

Vogt, M. 1954. The concentration of sympathin in different parts of the central nervous systems under normal conditions and after the administration of drugs. *J. Physiol.* (Lond.) 123:451.

Volicer, L., Scheer, E., Hilse, H., and Visweswaram, D. 1968. Turnover of norepinephrine in the heart during experimental hypertension in rats. *Life Sci.* 7:525.

von Euler, U. S. 1956. *Noradrenaline.* Springfield, Ill.: Charles C Thomas.

———, Hellner, S., and Burkhold, A. 1954. Excretion of noradrenaline in urine in hypertension. *Scand. J. Clin. Lab. Invest.* 6:54.

Wall, P. D., and Davis, G. D. 1951. Three cerebral cortical systems affecting autonomic function. *J. Neurophysiol.* 14:507.

Wang, S. C., and Ranson, S. W. 1939. Autonomic responses to electrical stimulation of the lower brain stem. *J. Comp. Neurol.* 71:437.

Ward, A. A., Jr. 1948. The cingular gyrus: Area 24. *J. Neurophysiol.* 11:13.

Weinberger, M. H., Dowdy, A. J., Nokes, G. W., and Leutscher, J. A. 1968. Plasma renin activity and aldosterone secretion in hypertensive patients during high and low sodium intake and administration of diuretic. *J. Clin. Endocrinol. Metab.* 28:359.

Weiner, H. 1970. Psychosomatic research in essential hypertension: retrospect and prospect. *Bibl. Psychiatr.* 144:58.

———, Singer, M. T., and Reiser, M. F. 1962. Cardiovascular responses and their psychological correlates. A study in healthy young adults and patients with peptic ulcer and hypertension. *Psychosom. Med.* 24:477.

Weiss, E. 1942. Psychosomatic aspects of hypertension. *J.A.M.A.* 120:1081.

——— 1957. *Psychosomatic Medicine,* 3rd ed., edited by E. Weiss and O. S. English. Philadelphia: Saunders.

Welch, A. S., and Welch, B. L. 1968a. Effect of stress and p-chlorophenylalanine upon brain serotonin, 5-hydroxyindoleacetic acid and catecholamines in grouped and isolated mice. *Biochem. Pharmacol.* 17:699.

——— and ——— 1968b. Reduction of norepinephrine in the lower brainstem by psychological stimulus. *Proc. Nat. Acad. Sci. USA* 60:478.

Welch, B. L. 1967. Aggression and defense: Neural mechanisms and social patterns. In *Brain Function,* edited by C. D. Clemente and D. B. Lindsley. Los Angeles: University of California Press.

——— and Welch, A. S. 1965. Effect of grouping on the level of brain norepinephrine in white swiss mice. *Life Sci.* 4:1011.

——— and ——— 1966. Graded effect of social stimulation upon d-amphetamine toxicity, aggressiveness and heart and adrenal weight. *J. Pharmacol. Exp. Ther.* 151:331.

——— and ——— 1968c. Differential activation by restraint stress of a mechanism to conserve brain catecholamines and serotonin in mice differing in excitability. *Nature* 218:575.

——— and ——— 1969. Aggression and the biogenic amines. In *Biology of Aggressive Behavior,* edited by S. Garattini and E. B. Sigg. Amsterdam: Excerpta Medica.

——— and ——— 1971. Isolation, reactivity and aggression: evidence for an involvement of brain catecholamines and serotonin. In *The Physiology of Aggression and Defeat,* edited by B. E. Eleftheriou and J. P. Scott. New York: Plenum.

Wenger, M. A., Clemens, T. L., and Coleman, D. R. 1961. Autonomic response specificity. *Psychosom. Med.* 23:185.

White, B. V., Jr., and Gildea, E. F. 1937. "Cold pressor test" in tension and anxiety: A cardio-chronographic study. *Arch. Neurol. Psychiatry* 38:914.

Whyte, H. M. 1958. Body fat and blood pressure of natives in New Guinea: reflections on essential hypertension. *Aust. Ann. Med.* 7:36.

Widimsky, J., Fejfarová, M. H., and Fejfar, Z. 1957. Changes of cardiac output in hypertensive disease. *Cardiology* 31:381.

Williams, G. H., Rose, L. I., Dluhy, R. G., McCaughin, D., Jagger, P. I., Hickler, R. B., and Lauler, D. P. 1970. Abnormal responsiveness of the renin aldosterone system to acute stimulation in patients with essential hypertension. *Ann. Intern. Med.* 72:317.

Williams, R. B., Jr., and McKegney, F. P. 1965. Psychological aspects of hypertension: I. The influence of experimental variables on blood pressure. *Yale J. Biol. Med.* 38:265.

———, Kimball, C. P., and Williard, H. N. 1972a. The influence of interpersonal interaction on diastolic blood pressure. *Psychosom. Med.* 34:194.

———, Lamprecht, F., and Lopin, I. J. 1972b. Serum dopamine-β-hydroxylase levels during development of various forms of hypertension in rats. *J. Clin. Invest.* 51:104a.

Wilson, C. 1961. Etiological considerations in essential hypertension. In *Hypertension—Recent Advances: The Second Hahnemann Symposium on Hypertensive Disease*, edited by A. N. Brest and J. H. Moyer. Philadelphia: Lea & Febiger.

Wilson, J. M. G. 1958. Arterial blood pressure in plantation workers in North East India. *Br. J. Prev. Soc. Med.* 12:204.

Wing, L. M. H., and Chalmers, J. P. 1974. Effects of p-chlorophenylalanine on blood pressure and heart rate in normal rabbits and rabbits with neurogenic hypertension. *Clin. Exp. Pharmacol. Physiol.* 1:219.

Winkelstein, W., Jr., and Kantor, S. 1967. Some observations on the relationships between age, sex, and blood pressure. In *The Epidemiology of Essential Hypertension*, edited by J. Stamler, R. Stamler, and T. N. Pullman. New York: Grune & Stratton.

———, ———, Ibrahim, M., and Sackett, D. L. 1966. Familial aggregation of blood pressure: preliminary report. *J.A.M.A.* 195:848.

Wise, B. L., and Ganong, W. F. 1960. Effect of brain-stem stimulation on renal function. *Am. J. Physiol.* 198:1291.

Wolf, S., and Wolff, H. G. 1951. A summary of experimental evidence relating life stress to the pathogenesis of essential hypertension in man. In *Essential Hypertension*, edited by E. T. Bell. Minneapolis: University of Minnesota Press.

———, Pfeiffer, J. B., Ripley, H. S., Winter, O. S., and Wolff, H. G. 1948. Hypertension as reaction pattern to stress: Summary of experimental data on variations in blood pressure and renal blood flow. *Ann. Intern. Med.* 29:1056.

———, Cardon, P. V., Jr., Shephard, E. M., and Wolff, H. G. 1955. *Life Stress and Essential Hypertension*. Baltimore: Williams and Wilkins.

Wolff, H. G. 1953. *Stress and Disease*. Springfield, Ill.: Charles C Thomas.

Wotman, S., Mandel, I. D., Thompson, R. H., Jr., and Laragh, J. H. 1967. Salivary electrolytes and salt taste thresholds in hypertension. *J. Chronic Dis.* 20:833.

Wurtman, R. J., Altschule, M. D., and Holmgren, U. 1959. Effects of pinealectomy and of a bovine pineal extract in rats. *Am. J. Physiol.* 197:108.

———, ———, Greep, R. O., Falk, J. L., and Grave, G. 1960. The pineal gland and aldosterone. *Am. J. Physiol.* 199:1109.

Yamori, Y., Lovenberg, W., and Sjoerdsma, A. 1970. Norepinephrine metabolism in brainstem of spontaneously hypertensive rats. *Science* 170:544.

Yankopolous, N. A., Davis, J. O., Kliman, B., and Peterson, R. E. 1959. Evidence that a humoral agent stimulates the adrenal cortex to secrete aldosterone in experimental secondary hyperaldosteronism. *J. Clin. Invest.* 38:1278.

Youmans, P. L., Green, H. D., and Denison, A. B., Jr. 1955. Nature of the vasodilator and vasoconstrictor receptors in skeletal muscle of the dog. *Circ. Res.* 3:171.

Zanchetti, A., and Zoccolini, A. 1954. Autonomic hypothalamic outbursts elicited by cerebellar stimulation. *J. Neurophysiol.* 17:475.

Zeaman, D., and Smith, R. W. 1965. Review of some recent findings in human cardiac conditioning. In *Classical Conditioning: A Symposium,* edited by W. F. Prokasy. New York: Appleton-Century-Crofts.

Zehr, J. E., and Feigl, E. O. 1973. Suppression of renin activity by hypothalamic stimulation. *Circ. Res.* 32(Suppl. I):I–17.

Zinner, S. H., Levy, P. S., and Kass, E. H. 1971. Familial aggregation of blood pressure in childhood. *N. Engl. J. Med.* 284:401.

INDEX

B

BEREAVEMENT
  and essential hypertension, 28
BIOFEEDBACK, and blood pressure, 40
BLOOD FLOW, and hypertension, 37–38
BLOOD PRESSURE
  adrenocortical disease and, 69
  age and, 22
  aldosterone and, 70–72
  angiotension and, 62–63
  conditioning studies and, 39–52
  coronary disease and, 31
  corticoids and, 72–74
  dopamine B(beta)-hydroxylase level,
    35, 44, 46, 49, 51, 74
  genetic factors and, 17–20, 47–51
  hypertension and, 15, 17
  kidney and, 57–63
  oral contraceptives and, 19
  pain and, 34–35, 38
  Personality and, 29–32
  prostaglandins and, 63
  psychophysiological factors in, 24–41
  renin and, 58–63
  salt and, 22–23, 66–67
  socioeconomic factors in, 22–24
  stress and, 16, 18, 23–24, 25, 39, 41
BRAIN
  and antidiuretic hormone, 68–69
  and blood pressure, 49–51, 80, 81–86
  and essential hypertension, 44–47

C

CARBOHYDRATE, intolerance to, 14
CARDIOVASCULAR SYSTEM, and essential
  hypertension, 53–57
CALCIUM
  and hypertension, 55–56
CATECHOLAMINES
  and essential hypertension, 74–77, 83
  and stress, 35, 50

CENTRAL NERVOUS SYSTEM
  and blood pressure control, 77–86
  and essential hypertension, 77–86
CHILDREN
  essential hypertension and, 30–31,
    33–34
CHLOROTHIAZIDE, and salt, 64
CIRCULATION, and essential hypertension,
  53–57 ·
CONDITIONING, cardiovascular response,
  39–52
CONN'S SYNDROME, 14, 69
CONTRACEPTIVES, ORAL, and high blood
  pressure, 19, 65, 78
CORONARY ARTERY DISEASE, and
  personality type, 31
CORTISOL, and high blood pressure,
  72–74
CORTISONAL, and hypertension, 56

D

DEPRESSION, blood pressure and, 30
DESOXYCORTICOSTERONE, blood pressure
  and, 69, 72–74
DIET, and high blood pressure, 22–23
DIURESIS, OSMOTIC, and angiotension,
  61–62
DOPAMINE β-HYDROXYLASE (DBH), and
  hypertension, 35

E

EPIDEMIOLOGY, of essential hypertension,
  20–22
EPINEPHRINE, and hypertension, 45–46
EXERCISE, and high blood pressure, 22

G

GENETIC FACTORS, in essential
  hypertension, 17–20, 33

124

PHENYLETHANOLAMINE
N-METHYLATRANSFERASE, and
essential hypertension, 145
PINEAL GLAND, and aldosterone secretion,
70
PITUITARY, and hypertension, 48
POTASSIUM
and aldosterone, 69−70
and 18-hydroxy-desorycorticosterone,
74
PROGESTERONE, and salt intake, 73
PROSTAGLANDINS
and blood pressure, 63
and corticoids, 72
PSYCHOPHYSIOLOGICAL FACTORS, in
essential hypertension, 24−41
PYELONEPHRITIS, and high blood pressure,
22

and desoxycorticosterone, 73
and peripheral resistance, 55−56
and water metabolism, 63−69
SEROTONIN, and hypertension, 45−46, 50
SODIUM
and aldosterone, 69−70
and angiotensin, 61−63
and blood pressure, 63−69
and hypertension, 55
and progesterone, 73
and renin release, 59
see also SALT
SOCIOECONOMIC FACTORS
in blood pressure, 22−24
in essential hypertension, 16−17,
22−24
STRESS
catecholamine level and, 35, 50
and hypertension, 16, 21, 23−24, 25,
28−34, 39, 41

R

REJECTION, and essential hypertension, 25
RENIN
and blood pressure, 71
and 18-hydroxy-desoxycorticosterone,
74
and hypertension, 14, 16, 17, 20, 48,
58−61
RESERPINE, and blood pressure, 75

T

TERRITORY, and high blood pressure, 44
TYROSINE HYDROXYLASE, and
hypertension, 45

V

VAGUS NERVE, and aldosterone secretion,
70
VASOCONSTRICTION
in conditioning studies, 39−40
and hypertension, 54−57
and pain, 35

S

SALT
and aldosterone levels, 50
and blood pressure, 18, 20, 22−23,
26−27, 47, 50−52